How Ordinary People Make Aid Work

How Ordinary People Make Aid Work

Civic Engagement and Health Aid Effectiveness

Stefan Kruse

JOHNS HOPKINS UNIVERSITY PRESS   BALTIMORE

Johns Hopkins University Press
2715 North Charles Street
Baltimore, Maryland 21218
www.press.jhu.edu

Library of Congress Cataloging-in-Publication Data is available.

A catalog record for this book is available from the British Library.

ISBN 978-1-4214-5254-8 (paperback)
ISBN 978-1-4214-5255-5 (ebook)

Special discounts are available for bulk purchases of this book. For more information, please contact Special Sales at specialsales@jh.edu.

EU GPSR Authorized Representative
ÐOGOS EUROPE
9 rue Nicolas Poussin
17000, La Rochelle, France
Email: contact@logoseurope.eu

To Sara and Mattea

Contents

Figures

Tables

Appendix Figures

List of Appendix Figures found in online supplement

Appendix Tables

List of Appendix Tables found in online supplement

How Ordinary People Make Aid Work

1

Participation in Health Development

External support can be useful as the oil that lubricates the engine of associational life, but it can never substitute for the hand that drives the car.

Michael Edwards, *Civil Society*, 2020

Effective development assistance can help save lives. Between 1990 and 2015, donors directed over US$500 billion toward health-care interventions in low- and middle-income countries (Dieleman et al. 2015). During this period, over one billion people were lifted out of poverty (World Bank 2018).[1] Central to donors' efforts to improve public health has been the empowerment of "the poor" through participatory innovations (Fung and Wright 2003). It was assumed that by creating spaces for citizens to express their voice, public institutions would become more responsive, contributing to broader development and democratic governance outcomes.

Merely creating opportunities for participatory activities, however, does not ensure accountability. Much depends on how beneficiaries engage with the provided opportunities (Cornwall 2008, 275). If individuals lack the resources to stand up against powerful interests or have no sense of belonging to a community, they may have little interest in spending time on "community" affairs. Citizens may also not be willing to participate in monitoring or evaluating service delivery if providers and officials are perceived as unresponsive (Hernández et al. 2019).[2] Available opportunities to exercise voice thus do not guarantee that citizens will be willing and able to hold officials accountable. Instead, citizen demand for accountability is shaped by the incentives that cultural and political context factors create. Donors, however, have paid little attention to the conditions shaping beneficiaries' actual willingness and capacity to participate in "invited spaces." In fact, despite more than three decades of support in international development for greater citizen participation, the aid effectiveness literature has almost entirely ignored how the cultural and political context shapes citizens' demand for accountability.

How Ordinary People Make Aid Work holds that a culture of civic engagement is vital for the success of development interventions aimed at improving population health. It asserts that participation in community organizations and social movements provides the resources and motivation that make citizens more likely to be mobilized into "invited spaces." Civic engagement is thus expected to empower beneficiaries to engage with providers and public authorities and to demand accountability. This book further argues that formal political institutions also have a role to play. High state capacity, democratic oversight institutions, and the devolution of power to the local level are expected to increase citizen demand and strengthen the impact of civic engagement on aid effectiveness.

Diverging from the literature on "invited participation," *How Ordinary People Make Aid Work* centers on spaces that people create for themselves (Cornwall 2008, 275). The focus lies on the impact of citizens' involvement in social and political groups that act independently and sometimes even in opposition to the government or external agencies. The book is not about the effectiveness of participatory projects or institutionalized governance mechanisms orchestrated by governments or international agencies, which has been addressed elsewhere (Mansuri and Rao 2013; Speer 2012; Falleti and Cunial 2018). The main interest lies in the role of autonomous citizen participation and how it empowers citizens to demand accountability in projects funded by development assistance for health, including aid that is not labeled "participatory" or "community driven." Such interventions are expected to be more successful in communities that have endogenously developed mechanisms for collective action and conflict resolution, facilitating effective demand for accountability.

Drawing upon evidence from studies on political participation, social capital, and citizen-led accountability, the book aims to uncover the conditions that bolster citizen demand and enhance aid effectiveness in the health sector. Herein, it offers several unique contributions: First, while the link between civic engagement and political action is a well-established finding in political culture research (Almond and Verba 1993; Verba et al. 1993;

Brady, Verba, and Schlozman 1995), this study is the first that tests its implications for the effectiveness of development assistance on a comparative basis. This fills a gap in the existing (macrocomparative) literature on foreign aid that almost exclusively centers on formal institutions. Beyond that, it deepens our understanding of political behavior and the importance of social capital in developing countries to improve public-service performance (Putnam 1993; Ostrom 1990, 1999; Paxton 2002, 2007).

Second, the analysis offers a nuanced assessment of the cultural and institutional determinants of accountability in public-service delivery and identifies systematic patterns of interaction between health aid, citizen participation, and formal political institutions. By assessing the effectiveness of health interventions across diverse contexts, the book also sheds light on public health's integral role in economic and political development, contributing to the broader field of comparative politics (Lipset 1960; Inglehart and Welzel 2005; Dyson 2013).

Third, *How Ordinary People Make Aid Work* employs the latest available data on global health financing and international public opinion from a broad sample of aid recipient countries spanning more than two decades. Employing dynamic panel data estimation and multilevel analyses, it addresses concerns related to endogeneity at both the individual and country level. The quantitative approach generalizes previous findings from qualitative and experimental research and details the impact of citizen participation under country-specific context conditions. From a practitioner's perspective, the book emphasizes that community relations shape health systems and provides insights into the type of civic involvement donors should prioritize in different political contexts.

Citizen Participation in Development Discourse

Donors provide development assistance for different purposes, often rooted in varied assumptions and theories of change (Lancaster 2006, 13–21). Historically, the promotion of development as a major purpose of aid has been both a means and an end of foreign policy. During the 1960s, for instance, development assistance came to be viewed as a means to promote democracy (Lipset 1959). Beyond strategic objectives, however, advancing development in impoverished nations has also been an end in itself, reflecting donors' commitment to altruism, social justice, and international solidarity (Lancaster 2006, 14). The thinking about foreign aid's role in promoting development significantly changed during the second half of the 20th century, as did the composition and allocation of aid toward public health and poverty reduction. Between 1990 and 2014, international health funding surged from $6.9 billion to $35.9 billion annually (Dielemann et al. 2015, 2361). This rise in health aid has quintupled the resources to improve service delivery through better-skilled health personnel, access to medical products and technologies, and improved administrative and management capacities for greater oversight of health-care providers. Yet, donor priorities have shifted over time, and different approaches to health development have placed varying degrees of importance on community involvement.

In the 1960s, the primary goal of development cooperation was economic development and material welfare. Therefore, foreign aid was mainly spent on industrial and infrastructure projects such as roads and dams, assuming that capital and technology transfer would create growth, which in turn was expected to reduce poverty.[3] In accordance with this view, the dominant theoretical perspectives on health and illness were based on technological magic bullets and biomedical models of health care, deemphasizing social, cultural, and environmental factors (WHO 2003, 139; Birn et al. 2009, 133). Correspondingly, international health agencies prioritized curative services based on high-technology and cost-intensive medicine and focused on (selective) disease-specific interventions. Community development and participation didn't play a major role as it was widely perceived as having failed during the first wave of participatory development in the 1950s (Mansuri and Rao 2013, 24–25).

In the 1970s, Western donors and multilateral organizations started questioning the expected trickle-down effects of economic growth. Based on the experiences of China, a consensus emerged that economic growth does not necessarily translate into better health for all but rather for those who are already better off, increasing the disparity in health status between the rich and the poor (Hsiao and Liu 1996). Thus, the importance of redistributive, pro-poor policies increasingly moved center stage. The focus of foreign aid shifted from economic growth to basic needs and the root causes of poverty.[4] Socioecological approaches thereby emphasized the importance of political, social, and cultural factors in understanding health and illness. Moreover, behavioral (learning) models viewed health primarily as a consequence of individual actions and beliefs that can be influenced by health education, counseling, and setting individual incentives (WHO 2003, 140).

As a result, the capital-centered view on development was gradually displaced by more people-centered approaches of development (Oakley 1991, 2). This is best illustrated by Article 5 of the UN General Assembly Resolution 2542 passed in 1969, which calls for "the active participation of all elements of society, individually or through associations, in defining and in achieving the common goals of development" (cited in Cornwall 2006, 70). There was also growing consensus that developing countries should prioritize prevention-oriented primary health care instead of high-tech and cost-intensive medicine (Tulchinsky and Varavikova 2009, 63). The Alma-Ata Declaration on Primary Health Care in 1978 reflects this shift in international health agencies' priorities from a narrow, medicalized approach to a holistic, people-centered approach, which integrates both technical solutions and the underlying social, economic, and cultural causes of ill health (Birn et al. 2009, 79). The declaration also asserted health as a fundamental right to all members of a society and emphasized that citizens have the right and duty to participate in the planning and implementation of their health care (WHO 1978). Moreover, the declaration considered community action to reduce health risks equally important as medical practitioners and institutional care (Tulchinsky and Varavikova 2009, 64). Furthermore, the World Health Organization (WHO) introduced the concept of community involvement in health development (CIH), which sought to include people in the decisions and actions that affect their health and prevent externally promoted health programs that do not meet the needs as defined by local communities (Oakley 1991, 12–49). Donors thus paid increasing attention to beneficiary involvement in the design and implementation of health programs. At the same time, a growing literature began challenging the view that individual self-interest undermines the effectiveness of voluntary organizations, as argued in *The Logic of Collective Action* by Mancur Olson (1965) and in "The Tragedy of the Commons" by Garrett Hardin (1968). As a result, donors have put more emphasis on communities' capacity and motivation to solve collective-action problems and the instrumental role of community-based organizations to enable participation and improve service delivery (Uphoff 1992, 326–387).

Despite reducing inequality in population health, the community-based, comprehensive primary-care approach was soon criticized for being unattainable because of the high costs and numbers of trained personnel required (Haines et al. 2007, 2121; Starfield, Shi, and Macinko 2005, 457). In their seminal paper, Walsh and Warren (1979) argued that a selective primary health-care approach addressing the few diseases responsible for the greatest mortality would be more cost-effective and, consequently, more appropriate for disease control in developing countries. Against this backdrop, many international health agencies became more supportive of selective interventions directed at medical solutions that de-emphasize the role of social, cultural, and political determinants of health. Moreover, the international debt crisis of the 1980s and the paradigm shift in economic theory led donors to stress the importance of reforming health systems for greater efficiency. The suggested reforms included introducing user fees and increasing competition from private-sector providers (Bennett 2011, 474). Thus, participation came to be viewed as a way to reduce the costs of development interventions by means of community contributions (Cornwall 2006, 72–74). At the same time, the World Bank and the International Monetary Fund provided structural adjustment loans to countries affected by the global economic crisis. These loans were coupled with a set of neoliberal policy reforms to "stabilize" the economy by reducing government spending and consumption, and expanding private-sector competition, decentralization, and the privatization of state-owned enterprises (Andrews 2013). The resulting large-scale reductions in public-health expenditures led to a significant decrease in the number of public employees delivering health (prevention) services (Birn et al. 2009, 80–85). Besides minimizing the role of the state and increasing citizens' choice (exit), the so-called Washington Consensus also encouraged donors to strengthen civil society's capacity to exercise pressure on service providers (voice). Enabling civil society to monitor elites and help social groups acquire the information, resources, and capacities necessary to hold governments, private contractors, and NGOs accountable became an integral part of donor activities (Brett 2003, 22).

The end of the Cold War provided legitimate ground for donors to assume that the Western model of state, market, and civil society is the best available blueprint for planning development in recipient countries. At the same time, a renewed interest among social scientists in the role of state institutions in enabling civil-society participation and shaping developmental outcomes placed the state back on the development agenda and has substantially influenced the way donors target aid (Evans, Rueschemeyer, and Skocpol 1985).[5] Democratic governance, economic liberalization, and freedom of association were viewed as inextricably intertwined (Cornwall 2006, 75). Elinor Ostrom's seminal work on the management of common-pool resources (1990) highlighted the ability of communities to effectively manage shared resources through institutional arrangements, including user associations, that enable cooperation and collective action. At the same time, the meaning of participation has expanded from engagement in community projects to engagement in the policy-making process and transformed participatory development into a means of mobilizing communities to monitor donor programs beyond individual development projects (Brett 2003, 4; World Bank 2000).[6] Attempts to strengthen citizens' capacity to monitor policymakers and service providers were complemented by efforts of the international community to build state capacity. As a result, donors focused on targeting both state institutions and civil society—often in the form of democracy assistance and as a strategy of aiding democracy abroad (Carothers 2011; van Rooy 2013, 31–70).

On the one hand, capacity-building exercises targeted public officials' values and attitudes, knowledge, and work ethics, aiming to improve government responsiveness (Eggen and Roland 2013, 30). Furthermore, new approaches were developed to enhance ownership and accountability, including sector-wide approaches (SWAps), debt-relief initiatives (HIPC), and poverty-reduction strategy papers (PRSPs).[7] With the ongoing privatization of public services, communities were encouraged to manage and provide their own services, shifting the meaning of ownership (Cornwall 2006, 75).

On the other hand, aid agencies recognized NGOs' ability to cooperate with community-based organizations that are closer to local culture (Banks, Hulme, and Edwards 2015, 708).[8] NGOs were considered instrumental in providing a wide range of (cost-effective) services and resources to membership-based organizations and those outside the reach of markets (Cornwall 2006, 74–77). NGOs also had a role in mobilizing political participation and empowering marginalized groups (Boulding 2014; Riddel 2013) as well as in the diffusion of norms and standards of gender equality (Paxton, Hughes, and Reith 2015; Paxton, Hughes, and Green 2006; Hughes et al. 2018).[9] Most donors focused on strengthening the organizational capacity of civil-society groups, investing in training, research, and policy work (van Rooy 2013, 64). As a result, NGOs became more numerous and received larger shares of development assistance from international donors (figure 1.1).

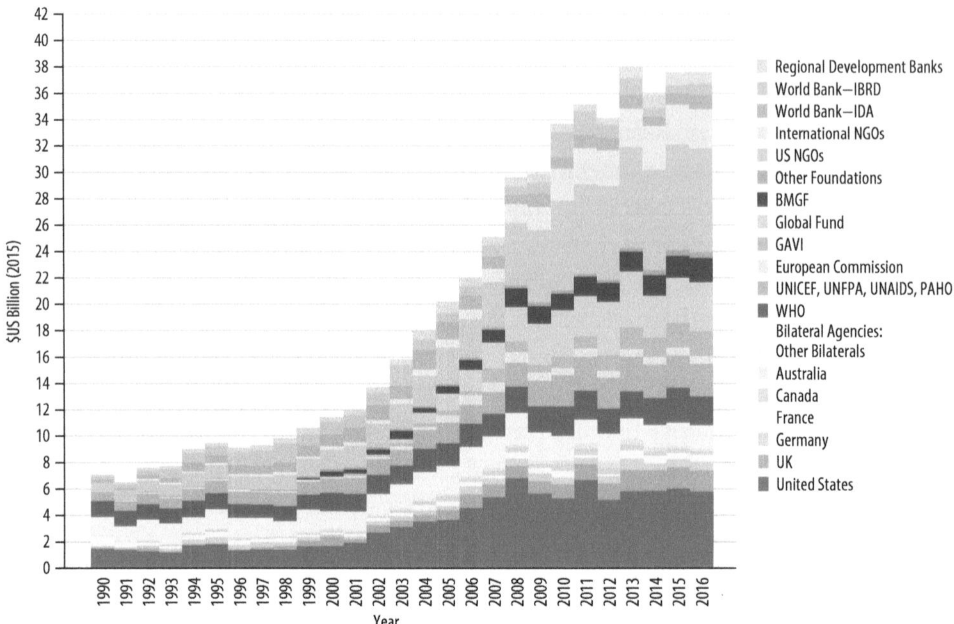

Figure 1.1. Health Aid by Channel of Disbursement (1990–2016). *Source:* IHME (2017).

The effectiveness of NGOs, however, has been questioned on several grounds. Critics have raised concerns about situations where NGOs inadvertently contributed to the fragmentation of health-service providers, and drained resources and staff away from health systems. Furthermore, the pressure to show tangible and measurable results to donors, and the limitations to impose sanctions against NGOs have also been cited to undermine NGOs accountability to beneficiaries (Kang 2010, 224; Riddell 2013, 379; Banks, Hulme, and Edwards 2015, 712; Winters 2010, 222–223). Parallel to these concerns, the situation in many recipient countries was characterized by "ubiquitous corruption of state officials, large gaps between the law and actual practice in business regulation, workers who do not even show up, doctors that do not doctor, teachers who do not teach" (Pritchett, Woolcock, and Andrews 2013, 1). In sum, the lofty expectations of simultaneously changing state institutions and civil society remained largely unmet. The growing skepticism toward the effectiveness of foreign aid led to the first decrease in total official development assistance provided by Western donors in the mid-1990s (DAC 2012, 266).

With the new millennium approaching, an international consensus emerged that poverty reduction requires global commitments, leading to the adoption in 2000 of the Millennium Development Goals (MDGs). Overall, foreign aid's annual growth rate increased from 5 percent in the 1990s to more than 11 percent after the international community adopted the UN Millennium Declaration (Dieleman et al. 2015, 2359).[10] In pursuit of the MDGs, donors allocated an increasing amount of foreign aid to the health sectors of the world's developing economies (figure 1.1). Specifically, the share of health aid in percent of total development assistance increased from 8 percent between 1990 and 2011 to 12 percent in 2014 (DAC 2016, 11). Since 1990, child and maternal health (MDG 4 and MDG 5) together received the largest share of funding (28 percent), followed by HIV/AIDS control (23 percent) (Dieleman et al. 2015). While in 1990 about 36 percent of health aid was provided for child and maternal health, funding for specific communicable diseases, such as HIV/AIDS, malaria, and tuberculosis, has increased considerably (figure 1.2).[11] In particular, funding for HIV/AIDS control increased by about 23 percent annually between 2000 and 2010, mainly fueled by the creation of the Global Fund and the United States' President's Emergency Plan for AIDS Relief (PEPFAR). Health aid for malaria and tuberculosis grew by about 26 percent annually, and together accounted for about 10 percent of health aid in 2010.

While donors increased their commitments to fight poverty, the work by Nobel laureate Amartya Sen has provided the intellectual underpinnings of a new approach for advancing human well-being that has strongly influenced development policy and practice (Sen 1999, 35–53; Evans and Heller 2015). Sen argued that "the people have to be seen . . . as being actively involved . . . in shaping their own destiny, and not just as passive recipients of the fruits of cunning development programs" (1999, 53). The approach was popularized by the United Nations Development Programme (UNDP) in its annual *Human Development Report* and focuses on improving people's lives and their opportunities rather than achieving higher incomes as an end itself (Haq 1995, 24–45). The *Human Development* approach emphasizes the importance of a broader set of factors contributing to human well-being, including health, education, and a decent standard of living. It also highlights the importance of people participating in the activities, events, and processes that shape their lives, and the complementary role of economic, political, and social institutions that enable participation (Haq

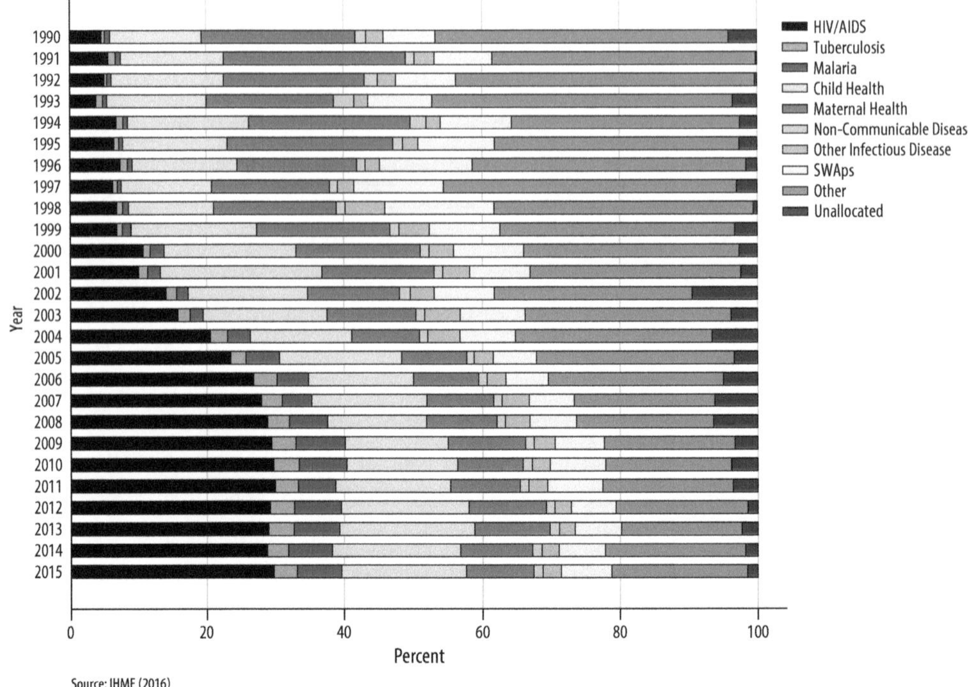

Figure 1.2. Focus Areas of Health Aid over Time (1990–2015). *Source:* IHME (2016).

1995, 13–23). These intellectual developments moved the concepts of empowerment and participatory development center stage and strongly influenced the policies and practices of international donors (Mansuri and Rao 2013, 29).

While institutional reforms failed in many recipient countries, donors continued their efforts to strengthen citizen voice and accountability to promote demand for better governance in recipient countries and to improve the quality of service delivery. The increased opportunities for citizen engagement with the state gave rise to a new generation of citizen-led, social-accountability action that aimed at enhancing the effectiveness of service delivery and improving the quality of democratic governance. The term "social accountability" refers to citizen-led actions that seek to hold the state to account, as well as efforts by the government, media, and other societal actors that promote or facilitate these actions (Malena and McNeil 2010, 1).

These new modes of citizen-led accountability action involve different mechanisms, including formal mechanisms (e.g., public-expenditure tracking surveys) and informal mechanisms of participation (e.g., social-movement activities). Citizen-led, social-accountability action came to be viewed as an especially relevant approach for societies where a representative government is weak, unresponsive, or nonexistent (Fox 2015, 246).

Alongside these changes, donor and recipient countries agreed upon reforming the existing aid system in the course of the international aid effectiveness agenda. In 2005, the Paris Declaration and the Accra Agenda for Action laid down fundamental principles to increase the effectiveness of foreign aid, including ownership, alignment, harmonization, managing for results, and mutual accountability.[12] Recipient countries were encouraged to set their own strategies to reduce poverty, tackle corruption, and build institutions. In turn, donors were called to align their interventions with national health priorities and use national health systems to deliver aid. As a result, many donors shifted focus to sector-wide approaches (SWAps) and health-sector support, with both growing by about 9 percent annually since 2000. For example, from 2009 to 2011, the World Bank channeled about half its resources to these areas.

With the life span of the MDGs coming to an end in 2015, the international community renewed its commitment to end poverty and adopted a new set of development goals as part of the 2030 Agenda for Sustainable Development. The Sustainable Development Goals (SDGs) shift the focus of international development efforts to the interdependencies between social, political, and environmental aspects while recognizing the importance of participation and cultural context.

The evolution of health-development paradigms over the course of more than half a century illustrates a trajectory toward greater participation and culture-based approaches to setting and working on development priorities (Badaan and Chaucair 2023, 236–238). Yet the new enthusiasm for participation has not been met with equally significant changes in development practices (Cornwall 2006, 78–79). Too little attention has been paid to the culturally embedded nature of the normative principles underpinning discourses of participation and the multifaceted causes of civic inertia that prevent the poor and marginalized from participating meaningfully in making the decisions that affect their health.

Plan of the Book

Addressing the contemporary debate about citizen participation and aid effectiveness, the first part of *How Ordinary People Make Aid Work* develops the theoretical argument. The second part of the book is empirical and describes differences in civic engagement, tests whether citizen involvement makes health aid work better, and explores the conditions under which this occurs. In particular, chapter 2 establishes the theoretical framework to assess the impact of civic engagement on health aid effectiveness in varying political contexts. Based on evidence from different strands of the literature, the chapter identifies when citizens in recipient countries exercise voice and demand accountability from providers and policymakers, highlighting the importance of both demand- and supply-side factors. Drawing upon these insights, the chapter develops a model that connects global health funding with improved population health via bottom-up accountability mechanisms and formal processes of top-down monitoring and horizontal oversight arrangements.

Chapter 3 describes the conceptualization and measurement of civic engagement, political institutions, and development assistance for health and provides an overview of the main methodological challenges in assessing the effectiveness of development assistance that characterize the current debate. The section further outlines the empirical approach and the estimation strategy chosen to assess whether civic engagement makes health aid work better and under which political context conditions.

Chapter 4 establishes the link between civic engagement and citizens' demand for accountability using international public-opinion data. The first part describes variations in social and political engagement across aid recipient countries. The second part examines to what extent differences in civic engagement are associated with communities' willingness and capacity to demand accountability based on citizens' interest in community affairs, democratic orientations and civic values, and adherence to cooperative norms. The last part compares how health aid and population health have coevolved within recipient countries of different civic-engagement levels.

Building upon the link between civic engagement and communities' willingness and capacity to demand accountability, chapter 5 answers the question of whether social and political engagement enhances health aid effectiveness. Precisely, the chapter tests whether an active citizenry that participates in voluntary activities and demands accountability through elite-challenging action makes development assistance for health more effective. A dynamic panel data analysis study looks at the combined effect of civic engagement and health aid on population health over the period 1990–2015. This study accounts for the simultaneity of aid allocation and aid effectiveness and considers endogenous sample selection. Furthermore, it compares the moderating effects of civic engagement with the effects of top-down performance oversight from state and democratic institutions. A multilevel-analysis study exploits variation within countries and examines the combined effect of civic engagement and health aid on self-rated health among individuals within recipient countries.

Chapter 6 proceeds to explore the institutional context conditions under which civic engagement influences health aid effectiveness. The chapter answers the question to what extent the moderating effects of civic engagement depend on recipient countries' political context. The main focus is on the interaction with formal political institutions that shape government responsiveness, including the role of state capacity, democratic oversight institutions, and decentralization of authority away from national governments. Chapter 7 elaborates on the key findings and relates them to the existing aid effectiveness literature. Furthermore, the chapter reflects on the generalizability of the results and summarizes the implications of the findings for research and the practice of development cooperation.

NOTES

1. The number of people living below the international poverty line (US\$1.90 in 2011 purchasing power parity dollars) declined from 1.9 billion people in 1990 to an estimated 736 million in 2015 (World Bank 2018). Yet, evidence from micro-level surveys of frontline service providers suggests that service delivery in many countries is still inadequate (World Bank 2017). For instance, between 1990 and 2010, Tanzania received US\$3.2 billion in health aid, yet by 2010, only 5 percent of its health facilities had access to electricity, clean water, or improved sanitation (World Bank 2012). Similarly, Uganda received US\$2.8 billion in development assistance for health between 1990 and 2013, but public health facilities faced widespread staff absenteeism, with personnel absent roughly half the time (Wane and Martin 2016). Comparable findings are reported in Molina and Martin (2016), Martin and Pimhidzai (2013), and Rockmore (2016).

2. By contrast, evaluations of community-based development projects have repeatedly shown that "invited participation" has the potential to enhance development outcomes depending on communities' collective-action capacity and the broader political context (Dasgupta and Beard 2007).

3. Economic development was explained using simple growth models, such as the Harrod-Domar model. According to this model, economic performance depends on a country's labor and capital stock, which in turn depends on investments and savings.

Consequently, development cooperation focused on closing the savings gap of developing countries by providing external resources for investment projects. Following this view, in the 1960s, the World Bank allocated about 75 percent of foreign aid to infrastructure projects (Thirlwall 1989).

Moreover, while economic development was the primary goal of development cooperation, modernization theory's claim that growth fosters democratization (Lipset 1959) provided further ground for achieving economic growth, especially in nondemocratic countries (Kruse 2023).

4. The "basic needs approach" was introduced by the International Labour Organization's World Employment Conference in 1976. The definition of "basic needs" included certain minimum requirements of a family for private consumption (such as adequate food, shelter, clothing, certain household equipment, and furniture) and essential services provided by and for the community, such as safe drinking water, sanitation, public transport, as well as health and educational facilities.

5. Following Douglass North, institutions are defined as a "set of norms that have a significant impact on the behavior of individuals" (1990). They shape how people act—either by fostering voluntary compliance with rules or by motivating behavior through the threat of sanctions. In this way, institutions create social order by aligning the expectations and actions of all actors involved (Lauth 2015, 57–58). In contrast to formal institutions, which are officially codified in written documents and derive legitimacy from rule-making authorities, informal institutions are "socially shared rules, usually unwritten, that are created, communicated, and enforced outside of officially sanctioned channels" (Helmke and Levitsky 2004, 727).

6. The mainstreaming of participation in development has a long history, ranging from the UN Resolution for active citizen involvement throughout the 1990s and 2000s through participatory and human development approaches as well as social capital and social accountability initiatives, to the adoption of the Sustainable Development Goals.

7. Poverty-reduction strategy papers (PRSPs) served as a mechanism to increase ownership and accountability by providing certainty for donor organizations that recipient countries will use aid to pursue development outcomes based on a jointly developed strategy. PRSPs also seek to promote citizen voice and the involvement of civil society in the design of aid programs. Sector-wide approaches (SWAps) sought to reduce duplication of service provision and donor fragmentation, whereas debt-relief initiatives (HIPC) aimed to free up resources for increased social spending. SWAps are usually supplemented with health-sector reforms such as decentralization and are often associated with delivering aid as budget support. For a critical discussion of SWAps and budget support, see Dijkstra (2013) and Molenaers, Dellepiane, and Faust (2015, 10).

8. Due to their heterogeneity, NGOs are broadly defined as nonprofit, voluntary organizations primarily focused on humanitarian objectives operating on a local, national, or international level (Kang 2010, 223–224). NGOs at different levels often cooperate through the exchange of funding resources, technical assistance, and joint program implementation. As intermediary and implementing institutions, they are active in training health professionals, providing technical assistance, and monitoring government services.

9. For instance, world polity theorists have argued that countries closely connected to the global net of international NGOs (INGOs) tend to adopt global practices and organizational norms, including those related to public-service funding or human-rights legislation (Paxton, Hughes, and Reith 2015, 287). Likewise, feminist-movement studies suggest the proliferation of women's international NGOs (WINGOs) has contributed to the spread of norms and standards of gender equality and increased international efforts to strengthen women's rights (Hughes et al. 2018).

10. Most of the contributions are channeled to bilateral agencies (about 40 percent) and NGOs and foundations (27 percent) (figure 1.1). Meanwhile, 14 percent is channeled to UN agencies, 13 percent to public-private partnerships, 9 percent to development banks, and 4 percent to the Bill and Melinda Gates Foundation (BMGF) (IHME 2016). The most important public-private partnerships include the Global Fund to Fight AIDS, Tuberculosis, and Malaria (GFATM) and the Global Alliance for Vaccines and Immunization (GAVI).

11. Across focus areas, a large part of health aid is used for training, including professional oversight and supportive supervision to improve the capacities of the health workforce (Miller et al. 2016). Over the period 1990–2013, international health funding for human-resource development amounts to about 4.8 percent. Estimates are based on the author's calculations using AidData (Tierney et al. 2011).

12. Increased ownership involves developing countries setting their own strategies for poverty reduction, improving their institutions, and tackling corruption. Based on these objectives, donors are expected to align their interventions with country priorities and use their local systems ("alignment"). "Harmonization" refers to coordination, simplification of procedures, and sharing of information to avoid duplication. "Managing for results" implies that developing countries and donors shift focus to development results and their measurement. "Mutual accountability" requires donors and partners to be accountable to each other for development results.

2

Participation, Accountability, and Aid Effectiveness

The impact of aid on development outcomes has been the subject of long-standing discussion. While proponents maintain that health aid improves service delivery, critics have questioned its effectiveness on many grounds. Positive outcomes have been highlighted in numerous studies. For instance, a recent study found that an aid inflow of 5 percent (of GDP) raises life expectancy by 2.4 years and reduces infant mortality by 14 deaths per 1,000 live births (Arndt, Jones, and Tarp 2015). Other studies emphasize foreign aid's role in reducing malaria- and HIV/AIDS-related mortality and enhancing the use of insecticide-treated nets (Hsiao and Emdin 2015; Bendavid and Bhattacharya 2009; Bendavid et al. 2012; Flaxman et al. 2010).[1] Counterevidence suggests, however, that health aid has failed to generally improve public health (Williamson 2008; Duber et al. 2010) and only benefits countries with low or moderate mortality rates (Kizhakethalackal, Mukherjee, and Alvi 2013). In high-mortality countries, however, its effectiveness has been questioned (Wilson 2011).

In light of these mixed findings, the debate has evolved from asking whether aid works or not to asking when aid is most likely to work (Glennie and Sumner 2016). Central to this is exploring the influence of recipient countries' specific context on the incentives embedded in development aid and the collective-action problems that donor agencies, public officials, and beneficiaries face (Gibson et al. 2005).

The following section outlines the concept of accountability as a useful framework to analyze the specific conditions under which aid improves the quality of service delivery and brings together evidence from both micro- and macro-level studies on participatory development and social accountability. It further spans research from the study of social capital, which focuses on the nature and extent of social interactions between communities and institutions, and provides important insights into the linkages between civic engagement, accountability, and political institutions in recipient countries. The concluding section synthesizes these findings, offering a framework and hypotheses to explore the specific context conditions that enhance the effectiveness of health aid.

Accountability in Development Projects

Service delivery problems often emerge from accountability gaps, a concept rooted in Alfred Hirschman's model of exit, voice, and loyalty (1970). In this framework, accountability largely depends on the availability of alternative service providers (exit) and the degree to which users can influence service outcomes through active participation or protest (voice) (Paul 1992, 1047–1048). By exercising voice, users can hold service providers accountable either directly ("short route" of accountability) or indirectly through policymakers and politicians ("long route" of accountability) (World Bank 2003). In aid recipient countries, however, citizens seeking improved service delivery are limited to directing their voice and accountability actions either at implementing organizations or their *own* government because of the geographical and political distance to donor governments.[2]

Recent efforts to strengthen beneficiary involvement in development projects and innovations in participatory governance have significantly increased opportunities for citizens to engage with organizational providers and public officials (Oakley 1991; Fung and Wright 2003).[3] These mechanisms enable citizens to participate in the planning, monitoring, and evaluation of service provision, express concerns to oversight institutions, or make financial or labor contributions that can be withdrawn if service quality decreases (Winters 2010, 221–232). Citizens may also participate in budgeting decisions or the monitoring of health policies in communities where formal mechanisms of participatory budgeting or municipal health councils exist (Falleti and Cunial 2018; Baiocchi 2003; Isaac and Heller 2003).[4]

At the same time, the rise of institutionalized modes of participatory governance has increasingly sidelined and undermined the legitimacy of traditional forms of citizen participation, including elite-challenging actions like protests and strikes (Cornwall 2008, 280–282). This proliferation of "invited participation" has thus limited the scope for people to set their own agendas, presuming that citizens are ready to engage with providers and officials (Cornwall and Coelho 2007, 5–10). Yet, in contexts where citizens are politically disengaged and deferential to elite decisions or where associational freedom and decentralized decision-making are restricted, participation is simply a pretence and remains ineffective (Oakley 1991, 10–14; Almond and Verba 1963; Pretty 1995).

The cultural and political contexts are even more important when citizens aim to hold implementing agencies, whether governmental or nongovernmental, indirectly accountable through policymakers and politicians. Governmental organizations' accountability to recipient governments, in particular, depends strongly on the effectiveness of state institutions and horizontal oversight mechanisms (World Bank 2003). Specifically, Weberian bureaucratic principles like hierarchical decision-making, meritocratic recruitment, and long-term rewarding career paths create incentives for officials, ensuring impartial, transparent, and effective service provision.[5] Democratic institutions further strengthen accountability through free and fair elections and the protection of citizen rights and media freedom. Independent oversight bodies such as anticorruption and electoral commissions further reinforce horizontal oversight within the state and electoral accountability of governments to voters, as highlighted by O'Donnell (1998).

In Costa Rica, for instance, the cultural and political context played a major role in the extension of basic health services to "the poor" and the subsequent rapid declines in infant mortality in the 20th century. In particular, McGuire (2010) attributes the country's improvements in population health to citizens' active involvement in community affairs, the spread of democratic values, and the country's long-term experience with democracy, including a free press and the freedom of assembly. Similarly, in countries like South Korea, democratic institutions coupled with technocratic state capacity have also enabled civil-society actors to demand accountability, leading to increased state responsiveness (Evans and Heller 2015).

The accountability of nongovernmental implementing organizations (NGOs) to recipient governments, on the other hand, is less influenced by political institutions owing to their nongovernmental nature and the limited opportunities for hierarchical oversight. Furthermore, the high international mobility of NGO personnel and the often-scarce information about their activities make direct oversight challenging. Nevertheless, funding as well as registration and reporting requirements remains an important mechanism to ensure that NGOs align with governments' (donors') policy agendas and priorities (Najam 1996, 342–343; Lewis and Kanji 2009, 26–29).[6] Hence, despite the weaker accountability relationship between NGOs and recipient governments, recent evidence suggests that NGO activities are associated with better population health, especially in countries with transparent democratic oversight institutions (McGuire 2020).

The Effectiveness of Foreign Aid

Whether aid is more effective in environments with greater accountability is the key question in the foreign aid literature. Various studies examine how political and macroeconomic contexts shape aid effectiveness at the country, sector, and project level.[7] While much of this literature centers on the impact of "institutional quality," there remains debate among practitioners and researchers regarding which institutional conditions are most important to enhance the effectiveness of foreign aid.

Previous research held that aid effectiveness depends on the quality of macroeconomic policies and state institutions (Burnside and Dollar 2000; Collier and Dollar 2002; Burnside and Dollar 2004).[8] More recent studies, however, challenge this view, demonstrating that neoliberal macroeconomic policies do not necessarily strengthen the effectiveness of aid (Easterly 2003). Findings from project evaluations remain inconsistent. Evidence from environmental aid projects, for example, suggests that government effectiveness plays an important role for better project outcomes (Buntaine and Parks 2013), while an evaluation of World Bank projects finds that institutional quality has no impact on project performance (Guillaumont and Laajaj 2006). Similarly, studies on health aid provide mixed findings, on the one hand suggesting that institutional quality strengthens the effectiveness of health aid (Mishra and Newhouse 2009), and on the other indicating that corrupt governments may effectively implement aid in certain sectors like health, where compliance is cheap, to attract additional aid inflows (Dietrich 2011).[9]

The aid effectiveness literature has also investigated the role of democracy. While initial studies failed to establish a link between political rights and aid effectiveness (Boone 1996), newer studies suggest that democratic institutions strengthen aid's impact on long-run economic growth and human development (Svensson 1999; Kosack 2003). Micro-level studies support these findings, showing that projects achieve better outcomes in countries where civil and political rights allow citizens to protest and demand accountability (Isham, Kaufmann, and Pritchett 1997, 236–237; Dollar and Levin 2005) and where beneficiaries participate in the implementation of development projects, giving beneficiaries not only voice but also the opportunity to withdraw their financial or labor contributions as a form of protest (Winters 2010, 232).[10] Evidence from the health sector, however, suggests that the presence of democratic institutions do not necessarily strengthen the effects of aid on population health (Wilson 2011).[11]

More recent findings indicate that democratic institutions can have differential effects on aid outcomes. Specifically, Wright (2010) demonstrates that personalist electoral rules, such as open-list proportional representation, create incentives for politicians to prioritize narrow, targeted spending over broad-based public-goods spending, diminishing aid effectiveness.[12] Conversely, electoral rules that prevent personalism in developing democracies strengthen the effectiveness of aid.

Another strand of the literature debates whether aid works better in decentralized recipient countries. The transfer of decision-making power, fiscal resources, and administrative competencies from central to local authorities is posited to give users more say in local service provision and to create incentives for providers to respond to local demands. While cross-country studies have yet to confirm that decentralization significantly enhances aid effectiveness (Lessmann and Markwardt 2012; Baskaran, Bigsten, and Hessami 2013), most health sector studies indicate that decentralization is linked to better service provision and significant improvements in child and maternal health outcomes (Segall 2003; Mogedal, Steen, and Mpelumbe 1995; Mansuri and Rao 2013, 207–212; Dwicaksono and Fox 2018). For example, Brazil's municipally managed Programa Saúde da Família (family health program) has reduced infant mortality by about 13 percent over a six-year period (Macinko et al. 2007). Further supporting this view, case studies from India, Argentina, and China also report positive health outcomes associated with increased subnational fiscal autonomy (Dwicaksono and Fox 2018; Jiménez-Rubio 2014; Uchimura and Jütting 2009).[13]

In summary, there is ongoing debate about how the context of aid recipients influences accountability between governments and citizens. The aid effectiveness literature has primarily focused on political factors, analyzing the role of state capacity, democratic institutions, and the level of decentralization. Evidence shows that neither sound macroeconomic policies nor high state capacity consistently improve aid outcomes. Aid tends to be more effective in countries with strong political and civil rights, yet electoral institutions that breed personalism can reduce governments' public-goods spending and weaken aid effectiveness. Furthermore, while subnational autonomy has little impact on aggregate aid effectiveness, it appears to strengthen the impact of aid on the quality of service delivery and population health.

In light of the mixed evidence, it is worth noting that many studies do not fully consider how aid may indirectly affect accountability and development outcomes by altering political institutions (Chauvet 2015, 359; Krasner and Weinstein 2014).[14] Moreover, the role of citizen participation, rooted in communities' capacity and willingness to engage in accountability action, is often overlooked, despite its potential to improve aid effectiveness (Baliamoune-Lutz and Mavrotas 2009; Baliamoune-Lutz 2012).[15] The lack of research on the impact of bottom-up mechanisms of performance oversight represents an important gap in the aid effectiveness literature, especially considering the growing consensus on the advantages of citizen engagement in accountability actions, which will be reviewed in the following section.

Citizen-Led Accountability Action and Service Provision

Citizen-led actions for accountability, also known as social-accountability initiatives, have spurred extensive research. They range from formal mechanisms like participatory public expenditure tracking to informal modes such as community-based monitoring of service provision (Peruzzotti 2011, 55).[16] Research consistently shows that the potential reputational and political costs to authorities and providers emerging from citizen engagement can lead to more responsive governments. In the health sector, for instance, citizen-led monitoring has been linked to decreased absenteeism among health-care professionals and improved health-service quality (Drèze and Sen 1995, 227–239; Björkman and Svensson 2009).[17] Citizen engagement can also increase political participation, raise citizens' awareness of their rights, and create more inclusive and cohesive societies (Gaventa and Barrett 2012; Joshi 2013).[18]

Increased citizen involvement may also contribute to greater corruption, elite capture, or state repression, however (Gaventa and Barrett 2012).[19] The impact of citizen engagement is influenced by various factors, including the availability of participatory spaces, citizens' motivation and capacity to occupy these spaces, and governments' openness to respond to citizen demands (Joshi 2013, 40; Carlitz 2013; Fox 2015), all of which are influenced by a country's political, legal, and historical context (Lodenstein et al. 2017). Accordingly, recent evidence suggests that an active civil society and programmatic political parties, along with state capacity, democratic oversight institutions, and decentralization, are crucial determinants of the effectiveness of citizen engagement (Hickey and King 2016; Brinkerhoff and Wetterberg 2016).

In summary, citizen-led accountability actions can significantly enhance government responsiveness and public-service quality. The impact of citizen engagement ultimately depends, however, on the societal and political context that shapes the vibrancy of civil society and the quality of formal oversight mechanisms. These findings align with the interdisciplinary study of social capital and state-society interactions, which will be further explored in the next section.

Social Capital and Public-Service Performance

Social capital reflects a way of conceptualizing how cultural, structural, and institutional aspects of small to large groups in a society interact and affect individual incentives and behavior and resultant economic and political change.

Elinor Ostrom and T. K. Ahn, "Social Capital and Collective Action," 2008

Social capital has played a pivotal role in international efforts to combat poverty and is recognized by the World Bank as a core element of empowerment and poverty reduction (UNDP 1993; World Bank 1994, 1998, 1999; Grootaert and van Bastelaer 2002). Highlighting the importance of social relationships in human behavior, social capital's influence extends beyond development studies, affecting research on democratic governance, public health, collective action, and environmental concerns (Woolcock 2010).[20]

The concept gained prominence in the social sciences through Robert Putnam's seminal study of community life in Italy and the democratic transitions in Eastern Europe and Latin America at the end of the 20th century (Putnam 1993; Stolle and Howard 2008). Putnam attributed Northern Italy's superior economic and governmental performance to its culture of civic engagement and trust, in contrast to Southern Italy's culture of "amoral familism," which limited citizen involvement and the extension of trust beyond closed in-groups. Drawing on the ideas of John Stuart Mill and Alexis de Tocqueville, he linked the observed differences in the vibrancy of associational life to communities' motivation and capacity to hold their governments accountable.[21] As Putnam puts it, "Citizens in civic communities expect better government and (in part through their own efforts), they get it. They demand more effective public service, and they are prepared to act collectively to achieve their shared goals" (1993, 182).[22] Nonhierarchical associations that connect people of different social background are thereby essential, as they foster out-group trust and respect for opposing views, and they strengthen citizens' skills and motivation to exercise voice (Fung 2003; Paxton and Ressler 2017).[23] Their role in bridging social divides, resolving conflicts, facilitating collective action, and improving democratic governance, economic development, and public health is central to debates among development researchers, practitioners, and policymakers (Grootaert and van Bastelaer 2002).[24]

Most studies support the neo-Tocquevillian view that civil societies' endowments of social capital are linked with increased democratic freedoms, reduced corruption, and greater government performance (Tusalem 2007, 379). Specifically, civil society's importance in curbing power abuses and promoting democratization is well documented (Schedler, Diamond, and Plattner 1999; Diamond 1999; Linz and Stepan 1996), with recent studies highlighting the democracy-enhancing effects of citizen engagement in mass movements (Hellmeier and Bernhard 2023). Furthermore, the positive relation between social capital and government responsiveness is well established (La Porta et al. 1997; Knack 2002; Bjørnskov 2010), although its impact on administrative efficiency is less clear (Andrews 2012; Tavits 2006).[25]

Contrary to the society-centered view, institutionalists hold that the development and effects of social capital depend on the broader institutional context (Rothstein and Broms 2012).[26] They warn that excessive mobilization of social forces can exacerbate social tensions and promote regime instability (Huntington 1968; Linz 1978).[27] Notable examples include the rise of the NSDAP in Weimar Germany (Berman 1997) and the Rwandan genocide (Armony 2004), where weak political institutions turned civil-society associations into a place for dissatisfied citizens and deepened existing cleavages (Berman 1997, 569–570).[28] The importance of institutions in building trust and overcoming collective-action problems is also evident in the management of common pool resources (Ostrom and Ahn 2008; Ostrom 1990, 1999).

Cross-national evidence supports the formative and conditioning effects of political institutions on social capital. Rothstein and Stolle (2008) highlight that generalized trust is closely linked to the impartiality of legal and administrative institutions. Further evidence suggests that formal democratic institutions are positively associated with interpersonal trust, democratic orientations, and civic engagement, including citizens' participation in elite-challenging actions (Paxton 2002; Roßteutscher 2010). The institutional context determines not only the formation of social capital but also its impact on public-service performance. A recent study across European regions reveals that civic engagement is more effective in reducing corruption in regions that lack transparent and merit-based institutions of bureaucratic governance (Larsson and Grimes 2022).[29] This is consistent with the finding that the impact of social capital on population health and economic growth is more pronounced in countries with weaker institutional quality (Knowles and Owen 2010; Ahlerup, Olsson, and Yanagizawa 2009). While both these findings imply that a lack of functioning state institutions can be substituted by social capital, the absence of democratic institutions cannot be compensated, weakening the impact of a vibrant civil society on mitigating corruption and resisting authoritarian rule (Grimes 2013; Roßteutscher 2010).

Theoretical Framework

This section synthesizes evidence from the literature on aid effectiveness, citizen action for accountability, and social capital to argue that a culture of civic engagement is essential for effective development interventions aimed at improving population health. It holds that participation in community organizations and elite-challenging actions provide the necessary resources and motivation for citizens to hold providers and authorities accountable and occupy "invited spaces" created by donor engagement. It further argues that the impact of community engagement is influenced by formal political institutions that shape government responsiveness and foster citizen involvement. The proposed model integrates citizens' demand for accountability and the role of cultural and political context factors to assess the effectiveness of health interventions in a comparative perspective.

Culture and Accountability Action

The importance of citizen participation for the success of development projects is widely recognized (Finsterbusch and Van Wicklin 1987, 1989; Narayan 1995; Winters 2010; Mansuri 2012). Effective participation in aid projects depends on citizens having access to understandable information about project outcomes, and their capacity and willingness to act on this information and engage with service providers and authorities.

In the health sector, for instance, access to information about the quality and quantity of service provision, its outcomes, and the role of elected officials is essential for citizens to hold providers and officials accountable (Goetz and Jenkins 2005, 58; Woolcock and Narayan 2000; Gibson et al. 2005). Critics, however, note that merely providing information is insufficient for effective performance oversight, highlighting the role of citizens' willingness and capacity to act on disseminated information.

Citizens who lack the resources to oppose powerful interests are unlikely to use relevant information, report corrupt officials, and activate formal accountability mechanisms (Ishihara and Pascual 2009; Lee 2011, 21). This challenges the implicit assumption of principal-agent models that ordinary citizens are willing to act like "principals" and enforce sanctions against corrupt behavior in service delivery (Fox 2015). From a human-empowerment perspective, communities' willingness to demand accountability largely depends on the availability of action resources and the spread of value orientations emphasizing the expression of shared concerns and equal opportunities (Inglehart and Welzel 2005; Welzel 2013; Welzel and Deutsch 2012). Resources empower people and enhance the social prevalence of values that encourage joint actions to keep elites honest, accountable, and responsive to citizens' needs (Welzel 2013, 37–56, 215–233; Welzel 2014; Welzel, Inglehart, and Klingemann 2003).[30] This modernization-based view is consistent with evidence from public health showing that value orientations and beliefs are critical to mobilizing citizen-led accountability action in health-service delivery (Cleary, Molyneux, and Gilson 2013).

Communities' motivation to demand accountability also depends on cooperative norms and individuals' expectations about whether others will participate in collective actions, like monitoring officials' behavior or imposing sanctions (Persson, Rothstein, and Teorell 2013).[31] According to this view, citizen demand for accountability is better conceptualized as a collective-action problem.

Communities' motivation to engage in accountability action is also influenced by the relational contexts in which people are embedded and the resulting societal expectations and behavioral norms (Markus and Kitayama 1991).[32] In more individualistic societies, where independence is valued, people put more emphasis on acting autonomously and pursuing one's own personal goals (Markus 2016).[33] This independent model of agency originates from (and reinforces) large social networks based on weak ties among people from diverse social backgrounds. Conversely, in more interdependent societies, individuals prioritize social obligations and collective goals, which stems from (and reinforces) small social networks based on strong ties within closed in-groups (Thomas and Markus 2023, 198–199). Individuals' motivation to participate in collective accountability actions is thus determined by the relational networks in which they are embedded (Markus 2016, 162). Consequently, citizens' associational involvement thus provides the connective resources that determine communities' capacity to engage in (collective) action and simultaneously shapes the relational forces that influence communities' willingness (Han 2009).[34]

In sum, while providers have incentives to suppress information that enables users to assess the quality of services, the presence of cooperative norms, action resources, emancipative values, and community ties provides the basis for communities' willingness and capacity to hold officials and providers accountable.

The Political Context of Accountability Action

The political context creates incentives that shape accountability through clearly defined rules and procedures, which ensures the capacity of states to maintain social order and improve public welfare, allows sanctioning of government ineffectiveness, and influences the willingness of public officials to be accountable to those they are supposed to serve. States' ability to implement and enforce, oversee, and transfer decision-making not only determines governments' responsiveness but also the impact of citizen participation in aid recipient countries, which is discussed in the subsequent section.

BUREAUCRATIC GOVERNANCE

State capacity is essential for public welfare and builds upon the state's ability to maintain social order and control within a nation's territory.[35] It involves making collectively binding decisions that are implemented with the appropriate organizational means and are normatively legitimized to ensure compliance (Genschel and Zangl 2014, 339). This capacity allows public officials to obtain, analyze, and disseminate relevant information, mobilize resources, and coordinate the provision of public goods with other providers (Loewenson 1998, 25–28).

State capacity can be conceptualized as a spectrum ranging from legal-rational authority to traditional authority (Weber 1947, 328).[36] The former relies on an organizational structure in which bureaucracies operate under the principles of impartiality, effectiveness, efficiency, transparency, and integrity (Norris 2012, 45). Bureaucratic governance is characterized by meritocratic recruitment, long-term rewarding career paths, hierarchical decision-making, functional specialization, and standardized procedures based on written documents that allow decisions and transactions to be reviewed (Weber 1978). Conversely, traditional authority relies on personal networks and corruption.[37] The recruitment of public officials in traditional states is based on patronage, and the delivery of goods and services relies on electoral clientelism.[38] In patronage states where public employment is allocated to reward loyalists, public officials tend to be poorly skilled, undermining the state's capacity to ensure the provision of public services and continuity in policy implementation (Norris 2012, 47).

Despite the importance of state capacity to set and communicate health-system priorities and monitor the achievement of policy goals, research on governance in areas of limited statehood indicates that a lack of state capacity does not necessarily lead to bad governance and ineffective service provision (Börzel and Risse 2010, 2016; Risse, Börzel, and Draude 2018). For instance, case study evidence from the Global Fund's malaria and tuberculosis project in Somalia shows that external actors can effectively deliver simple services in failed states, despite the state's lack of territorial control and enforcement capacity (Schäferhoff 2014). Similarly, Jennifer Murtazashvili's study on rural Afghanistan (2016) further illustrates how traditional (customary) organizations and trust can compensate for the limitations of weak state institutions, facilitating effective and legitimate governance and the provision of public goods and political order.

DEMOCRATIC OVERSIGHT

Numerous studies have explored the link between democracy and population health, most of them reporting a positive or null relationship (McGuire 2010, 2020; Gerring, Thacker, and Alfaro 2012; Mejia 2022; Gerring, Knutsen, and Berge 2022).[39] Unlike these studies, which focus on certain aspects of democracy and its direct impact on health outcomes, *How Ordinary*

People Make Aid Work views democracy as a context condition that enables ordinary citizens to make aid work better.[40] Accordingly, the focus lies on citizen power and how its impact varies between authoritarian and democratic environments.

Civil society's ability to exercise voice and hold officials and providers in recipient countries accountable largely depends on formal democratic institutions that create incentives for citizens to engage in oversight activities and for authorities to respond to citizen demands. In other words, the success of citizen-led accountability action depends upon whether freedom of assembly and the media is guaranteed, and whether effective horizontal oversight institutions exist (Blair 2011, 38). The role of independent judicial and legislative bodies is essential as they have the authority to prosecute illegal behavior and can be activated by civil-society organizations. A competitive multiparty system with ideologically diverse parties is likely to increase the likelihood of an opposition party taking up civil society's concerns in the legislature (Goetz and Gaventa 2001, 11). The impact of civic engagement is undermined, however, if court officials or legislators subvert official operating procedures in exchange for support from special interests or if governments suppress political opposition (Goetz and Jenkins 2005, 47–50).

Whether political leaders support or impede citizen involvement, in turn, depends on various factors, including the structure of government financing. Selectorate theory suggests that political leaders who rely on taxing economic activity to generate revenue are unlikely to curtail democratic rights and constrain citizen participation because repressive measures are likely to reduce economic activity too (Bueno de Mesquita and Smith 2009, 2010).[41] By contrast, leaders with access to free resources, such as foreign aid, can suppress democratic rights to reduce the threat of elite-challenging action with little impact on their revenue. Hence, if citizens demand accountability from governments that have access to foreign aid and are constrained by democratic institutions, selectorate theory predicts that political leaders spend the free resources on the provision of public goods. By contrast, in aid recipient countries without democratic oversight institutions, political leaders subject to the pressing demands of elite-challenging action are more likely to use the resources to curtail public-good provision and compensate coalition members with private goods (Bueno de Mesquita and Smith 2009, 2010).[42] Consequently, given the nature of government financing in aid recipient countries, democratic institutions create incentives that make governments more likely to respond to citizens engaging in elite-challenging accountability actions.

DECENTRALIZATION

Besides bureaucratic governance and democratic institutions, effective monitoring and oversight of service providers depend upon the distance between governments and end users and thus the extent of decentralization (Brinkerhoff and Wetterberg 2016). By devolving power and authority from central to local authorities, decentralization fundamentally changes the incentives faced by public officials and, thus, their behavior (Faguet 2014, 5). In centralized systems, public officials are usually selected by higher-level authorities of the central government, who have power over their salaries and professional prospects. In decentralized systems, public officials' tenure and career prospects are in the hands of the citizens they serve and who elect them (5). Thus decentralization incentivizes public officials to respond to local citizens' preferences as opposed to central governments' priorities.

Decentralization is also posited to foster democracy by strengthening citizens' participation in local governance, instituting regular elections, and improving access to information. Increasing citizen participation by way of decentralization enables service users to better articulate their needs and preferences to local representatives and better monitor local health-service providers and local governments. As a result, local officials and politicians are more open to public scrutiny (than national governments) and, hence, more accountable to the communities and individuals they are supposed to serve (UNDP 1993, 66–67). In the context of development assistance, public-service provision becomes more effective if the communities concerned have a real say in the planning and implementation. Furthermore, better informed local governments are more likely to allocate aid according to the needs of a heterogeneous population, increasing the efficiency of public services and thus aid effectiveness (Lessmann and Markwardt 2012, 1724–1725).

As public officials live closer to citizens, however, decentralization also creates more opportunities for corruption at local levels by making officials more often subject to the pressing demands of local interest groups (Prud'homme 1995; Bardhan and Mookherjee 2006; Tanzi 1996; Bardhan 2002). Specifically, staff in organizations may face conflicting incentives and pressures due to local contexts and informal institutions, including the influence of traditional authorities, which can weaken existing mechanisms of collective action. Decentralization can also produce confused responsibilities and impede coordination and cooperation if organizational mandates of elected politicians, chiefs, and city authorities are ill defined and overlapping. As a result, decentralization may cause policy incoherence and decision-making that directly conflicts with the resource planning of line ministries. Supporting this view, Lessmann and Markwardt (2010) find that fiscally decentralized countries without effective monitoring institutions suffer more corruption than non-decentralized countries.

Explaining Aid Effectiveness

Since the 1990s, donors have advocated for greater participation in development interventions, creating "invited spaces" to ensure that aid is more effectively targeted and implementing organizations are more accountable to local populations. The aid effectiveness literature, however, has overlooked how the cultural and political context of recipient countries shapes citizens' willingness and capacity to use the provided opportunities (Cornwall 2008). Citizens may have little interest in spending time on community affairs and engaging in accountability action if they have little sense of belonging to a community, lack action resources, or perceive local providers and public officials as unresponsive or corrupt.

Research on citizen-led accountability actions and social capital underscores the significance of community organizations and social movements that provide citizens with the necessary resources and motivation to engage in "invited spaces" (Mansuri and Rao 2013, 39). For the same reason, donors usually rely on established local organizations to sustain service provision beyond the lifespan of development projects (Kang 2010; Brett 2003; Dorsner 2004; Lewis 1998; Oakley 1991, 12–14). Evidence from development research also highlights the importance of an enabling political context and the role of formal oversight institutions.

Synthesizing these literatures, the following section summarizes how the cultural and political context shapes citizens' demand for accountability and determines the effectiveness of health interventions.[43] On the demand side, communities' capacity to engage in accountability actions depends primarily on the informational, connective, and material resources to voice their claims and engage in collective action, including the strength of community ties. Their willingness to demand accountability further relies on the spread of value orientations that emphasize the expression of shared concerns and equal opportunities, and individuals' expectations about the behavior of others.

On the supply side, effective oversight of service delivery in recipient countries requires autonomous actors who can coordinate with accountability actors (allies) within the state to impose sanctions. Central to this is the presence of civic space and linkages to the judiciary and legislative investigation commissions that have the authority to pursue legal action. Moreover, states' administrative capacity to implement policies, manage resources, and monitor the delivery of public goods is essential, as it feeds back into perceptions of social problems and shapes subsequent public demands (Norris 2012, 37). Insights from social-movement research underscore the significance of both democratic institutions to provide space for citizen action and effective government institutions to respond to citizen demands (Tilly 2006; Tilly and Tarrow 2015, 56–58). In environments with higher state capacity and democratic institutions, citizen action tends to be less violent and to have fewer adverse effects on public health.

Furthermore, better-informed local governments that have a real say in their planning and implementation are more likely to respond to the varying local demands, thereby increasing the efficiency of service provision (Lessmann and Markwardt 2012). As a result, service provision in aid recipient countries is more likely to be faster, better, fairer, more inclusive, and sustainable if public officials are held accountable through democratic principles and impartial, standardized administrative procedures—especially if officials and politicians are more open to public scrutiny due to the devolution of power to subnational levels (Arugay 2016, 7).

Against this backdrop, *How Ordinary People Make Aid Work* argues that civic engagement improves the effectiveness of development assistance for health. In particular, social and political engagement enables and motivates individuals to exercise voice, demand accountability, and directly engage in development projects. Correspondingly, development assistance for health (DAH) should be more effective in recipient countries with higher social and political engagement levels. To differentiate between more- and less-contentious modes of political participation, I further distinguish between elite-challenging political engagement, including attending a lawful demonstration, signing a petition, and joining a boycott, and all other elite-entrusting modes of political engagement. Hence, social engagement (Hypothesis 1a), elite-entrusting political engagement (Hypothesis 1b), and elite-challenging political actions (Hypothesis 1c) are expected to enhance the effectiveness of health aid in recipient countries, respectively. At the same time, the political context creates incentives that shape both citizens' demand for accountability and governments' responsiveness, conditioning the impact of civic engagement.

Institutions of bureaucratic governance ensure that public employment is allocated to highly skilled professionals, increasing the reliability of government decision-making. This better decision-making capacity and organizational competence enables bureaucratic states to better manage, implement, and monitor health system processes and respond to citizen complaints and recommendations that emerge from participatory development projects (Fox 2015, 353).

Bureaucratic governance further prevents health aid from being targeted toward narrow constituencies or allocated inefficiently, creating incentives that increase the prospects of citizen participation. In contrast, in patronage states with widespread corruption, citizens have little incentive to monitor public officials and voice their claims because of the high short-term costs of challenging corrupt practices. By implication, in recipient countries with higher bureaucratic governance, the enhancing effects of social engagement (Hypothesis 2a), elite-entrusting political engagement (Hypothesis 2b), and elite-challenging political activities (Hypothesis 2c), respectively, are expected to be stronger.

Effective monitoring and oversight over service providers is also closely tied to the independence of the judiciary and legislature, which have the authority to prosecute illegal behavior and can be activated by civil-society organizations. Democratic structures and processes, including free and fair elections and media autonomy, create incentives both for citizens to demand accountability and for politicians to respond. They also lower the individual costs of citizen participation, particularly in elite-challenging actions. Under democratic rule, beneficiaries may penalize poor service delivery and hold implementing agencies indirectly accountable through national governments and electoral mechanisms. Furthermore, democratic freedoms like access to information and freedom of association enable civil-society organizations to articulate demands and disseminate information on oversight outcomes.

Under democratic regimes that require broader support for political survival, political leaders confronted with elite-challenging mass movements are more likely to respond to citizen demands by using aid to provide public goods. Conversely, a lack of democratic institutions creates incentives for political leaders to reduce public-good provision and divert aid away to lower the threat that elite-challenging mass movements pose to leaders' survival (Bueno de Mesquita and Smith 2010). Consequently, the quality of democratic institutions is likely to condition the proposed synergistic effect of civic engagement. In more-democratic recipient countries, the enhancing effects of social engagement (Hypothesis 3a), elite-entrusting political engagement (Hypothesis 3b), and elite-challenging political actions (Hypothesis 3c), respectively, are expected to be stronger.

Effective performance oversight also depends on the presence of power-sharing arrangements. Decentralization increases citizens' choice (exit) between service providers and strengthens citizens' participation in local governance. Specifically, reducing the distance between governments and citizens enables service users to better articulate their needs and preferences to local representatives and better monitor local health-service providers and local governments. Devolving power and authority from higher to lower levels of government thus changes the local authorities' incentives and behavior. While public officials face strong incentives to respond to central government priorities, decentralization creates incentives for local officials to respond to those they are supposed to serve and by whom they are elected. As a result, local officials and politicians are more open to public scrutiny than national governments. Better-informed local governments are thus more likely to allocate aid according to the varying local demands of a heterogeneous population. Consequently, decentralization should enhance the effect of citizens' demand for accountability in aid recipient countries because it allows communities to have a real say in the planning and implementation of local development projects. By implication, the higher a recipient country's decentralization level, the stronger the enhancing effects of social engagement (Hypothesis 4a), elite-entrusting political engagement (Hypothesis 4b), and elite-challenging political activities (Hypothesis 4c).

To explore the cultural and political context conditions of accountability in service provision, this section derived a set of testable hypotheses about how civic engagement and political institutions condition the effectiveness of health aid in recipient countries. The next chapter outlines the measurement of the key concepts and discusses the methodological challenges associated with assessing aid effectiveness before laying out the empirical approach of this study.

NOTES

1. Further evidence suggests that the positive relationship between aid and population health tends to intensify over time (Bendavid and Bhattacharya 2014). It has also been shown to hold when controlling for factors like government health expenditures (Afridi and Ventelou 2013) and remittances from international migrants (Chauvet, Gubert, and Mesplé-Somps 2013).

2. In aid recipient countries, the long route of accountability is disrupted by the geographical and political divide between service users and voters. Even when service users observe donor organizations' performance in recipient countries, they cannot hold policymakers in donor countries accountable (World Bank 2003, 203–204; Gibson et al. 2005). Or as Bertin Martens puts it: "Foreign beneficiaries have no direct political leverage on donor country decision-makers. It is somewhat hard to see why donor country politicians would use voters' taxes to satisfy the needs and wishes of non-voters, unless voters have a stake in it too—that is, unless there is domestic demand for foreign aid transfers" (2002, 154).

3. In this context, accountability implies that citizens have the right to hold providers "to a set of standards, to judge whether they have fulfilled their responsibilities in light of these standards, and to impose sanctions if they determine that these responsibilities have not been met" (Keohane and Grant 2005, 25). According to this definition, accountability is a relationship between two parties: the demand side, which seeks answers and imposes sanctions, and the supply side, which is held accountable. It involves the obligation to provide information about what was done and explanations of why it was done (answerability), and it makes sanctions available for illegal or inappropriate actions (enforceability), including political sanctions, like voting someone out of office, and social sanctions, such as the loss of reputation.

4. In contrast to this study's focus on the conditioning effects of civic engagement, Falleti and Cunial (2018) examine the origins of participatory governance institutions in public health, focusing on health systems of Western Europe and Latin American countries. The authors argue that administrative governance reforms are likely to result in programmatic participation for monitoring, whereas political reforms due to regime or government changes are linked to the emergence of programmatic participation for policy-making (Falleti and Cunial 2018, 3–9).

5. In the health sector, for instance, effective state institutions ensure that the ministry of health monitors compliance with health regulations, sanctions noncompliance, and manages the contracts with implementing organizations that provide goods and services.

6. Yet critics have argued that the competitive nature of contracting nongovernmental implementing organizations creates incentives that can undermine NGOs' accountability to national governments (Winters 2010, 222–223). Others have highlighted that the effects of donor funding on the performance and accountability of nongovernmental implementing organizations ultimately depend on the specific context, including the relational forces that shape the potential for cooperation among the actors involved (Edwards and Hulme 1996, 969).

7. Here the focus is on the accountability relation between the government and its citizens in recipient countries. By contrast, aid effectiveness studies with a focus on the relationship between donors and recipient governments explore factors such as donor fragmentation, aid volatility, and aid dependency. Evidence from this literature suggests that aid is more effective if it is concentrated and stable because unpredictability and aid dependency make recipient countries more vulnerable to changes in donor behavior, like delayed or unpaid disbursements of funds (Glennie and Sumner 2016, 65–67; Lane and Glassman 2007, 941).

8. Several authors have replicated the original study of Burnside and Dollar (2000), demonstrating that the effectiveness of aid does not depend on certain macroeconomic and budgetary policies (Dalgaard and Hansen 2001; Easterly 2003; Dalgaard, Hansen, and Tarp 2004; Rajan and Subramanian 2008). At the same time, research on the developmental impacts of states' administrative and organizational capacities has broadened the focus of the aid effectiveness literature from policies to institutional quality (Evans and Rauch 1999; Fukuyama 2004). In particular, revisiting their previous study, Burnside and Dollar (2004) find that institutional quality (measured by the World Bank's Worldwide Governance Indicators) strengthens the impact of aid on economic growth. Despite this important study, there have been very few empirical attempts testing whether state capacity influences the effectiveness of aggregate aid flows (Chauvet 2015, 357; Wright and Winters 2010, 68).

9. Dietrich argues that countries with low administrative capacities are more likely to implement health aid effectively in order to signal compliance to donors and attract larger amounts of additional resources that can then be misappropriated for personal gain. Examining the interaction between corruption and health aid for immunization over the period 1990–2004, the author finds a negative relationship between the quality of institutions and health aid effectiveness.

10. The beneficial effects of citizen participation in the implementation of development projects have been shown across various sectors, including infrastructure (Mansuri 2012; Khwaja 2004; Finsterbusch and Van Wicklin 1987, 1989) and water supply and irrigation (Isham and Kähkönen 2002; Isham, Narayan, and Pritchett 1995; Narayan 1995, 21–52).

11. It is important to note that by selecting only high-mortality countries, Wilson's study (2011) explicitly excludes those democratic aid recipient countries that have experienced substantial improvements in population health.

12. Wright's study (2010) sheds light on the incentives to allocate aid that public officials face under different electoral rules. The author's findings indicate that electoral institutions, including open-list proportional representation, the absence of vote

pooling, multiple votes, and multiple ballots, create incentives for politicians to cultivate a personal vote, which makes them more likely to pursue corruption and target government spending to narrow constituencies, thereby decreasing aid effectiveness. By contrast, in democratic countries with lower levels of personalism, aid increases economic growth and public-good provision.

13. For a more comprehensive review of the literature on the outcomes of decentralization reforms, including evidence from OECD countries, see Dwicaksono and Fox (2018) and Jiménez-Rubio (2014).

14. For instance, aid can hinder the emergence of a taxation system, block democratic reform, and make recipient governments less accountable to their citizens. Moreover, aid can draw away talented bureaucrats from the government sector to work for international agencies and thereby weaken state capacity (Winters 2010). While several studies indicate that aid harms bureaucratic governance (Knack 2001; Bräutigam and Knack 2004; Rajan and Subramanian 2007; Busse and Gröning 2009), Tavares (2003) and Charron (2011) find that aid, especially multilateral aid, has significantly lowered corruption since the 1990s. Regarding the quality of democracy in recipient countries, most studies report a negative effect of aggregate aid (Djankov, Montalvo, and Reynal-Querol 2008; Kalyvitis and Vlachaki 2012) or no impact (Knack 2004). Aid for democracy promotion appears to bolster democratic quality (Kalyvitis and Vlachaki 2010; Dietrich and Wright 2013), however, especially if political leaders expect to remain in office after democratization (Wright 2009) or aid comes from democratic donors (Bermeo 2011).

15. Studies indicate that both ethnic fractionalization, as a proxy for social capital, and the absence of ethnic tensions, reflecting social cohesion, significantly boost the impact of foreign aid on economic growth (Baliamoune-Lutz and Mavrotas 2009; Baliamoune-Lutz 2012). Even though the authors do not spend much time explaining the underlying mechanisms, both findings are consistent with the view that the capacity of communities to engage in collective action and demand accountability enhances the impact of aid.

16. Formal mechanisms tend to mobilize already authorized publics to articulate their demands, while informal mechanisms are more likely to activate mute citizens and transform inertia into public action (Lee 2011, 22).

17. To identify the causal effect of community monitoring, Björkman and Svensson (2009) collected information on health providers' performance using citizen report cards. This information was disseminated at community meetings and contrasted with other providers' performance and government standards for health-service delivery. Communities were then encouraged to identify key problems and ways to monitor the health providers to improve health-service delivery. After the intervention, treatment communities were more involved in monitoring activities, which led to a significant reduction in staff absenteeism and waiting time and increased the use of health facilities, which in turn improved health-service quality and lowered under-five mortality.

A follow-up study further highlights the critical role of disseminating information about the status of health services in public facilities to enhance the effectiveness of community monitoring (Björkman Nyqvist, de Walque, and Svensson 2017; Björkman and Svensson 2009). The impact of information dissemination, however, remains disputed (Banerjee et al. 2010; Lieberman and Posner 2014; Keefer and Khemani 2016).

18. In one of the most systematic evidence-based studies, John Gaventa and Gregory Barrett classify the outcomes of citizen engagement based on 100 case studies across 20 countries. The authors classify the outcomes by mode of engagement, revealing that more than 90 percent of the outcomes linked to citizen engagement in local associations and over 70 percent from involvement in social movements were positively evaluated. By contrast, only about half the outcomes of citizen engagement in formal participatory governance spaces were rated positively.

19. Experimental evidence from Indonesia, for instance, demonstrates that community monitoring in road construction projects has little impact on the quality of service provision and corruption control (Olken 2007).

20. Evidence from public-health research suggests that associational membership, both at the individual and community level, significantly bolsters individual well-being (Kawachi, Kennedy, and Glass 1999; Putnam and Helliwell 2004; Kawachi, Subramanian, and Kim 2008). Yet the direct health effects of social capital are not the subject of this study.

21. Putnam defines social capital as "features of social organization, such as trust, norms, and networks that can improve the efficiency of society by facilitating coordinated actions" (1993, 167), conceptualizing it as a collective good (system capital) that benefits everyone, compared to social capital as a property of individuals (relational capital) (Inkeles 2000; Esser 2008). Individual social capital can be seen as the sum of all resources an actor can employ and use through personal relations with other individual actors who control those resources (e.g., their wealth, power, or reputation) and is reflected in the structure of actors' relations within a network. Like human or economic capital, the actor can intentionally invest in individual social capital and to a certain extent use it intentionally for personal gain. By contrast, Putnam views social capital as a collective community attribute, focusing on the structure of communities' entire system of networks.

22. Critics argue that the neo-Tocquevillian approach doesn't clearly explain how community collective action enhances government performance. Boix and Posner (1998) propose five potential mechanisms linking social capital and government effectiveness. First, active citizens, being well informed and engaged, critically assess government performance, demanding that political elites govern more effectively. Second, civic orientations and trust shape expectations about others' compliance with policies, reducing transaction costs and freeing up resources for improving public-service delivery. Third, social capital can change individual preferences toward community-oriented concerns, strengthening support for policies that benefit the whole community. Fourth, social capital can improve cooperation among bureaucrats, enhancing administrative efficiency. Fifth, social capital can help bridge social divides, enabling consociational democracy in divided societies.

23. Putnam underscores the importance of horizontally organized associations based on reciprocity and cooperation, in contrast to those organized hierarchically based on authority and dependency (1993, 88). This differentiation aligns with Mark Granovetter's seminal study on the strength of weak ties (1973) and the distinction between bridging and bonding social capital (Putnam 2000).

Bridging social capital is based on weak (inter-community) ties that bridge gaps between "closed" communities and increase access to nonredundant information.

Conversely, bonding social capital is based on strong (intra-community) ties, loyalty, and cohesion within closed in-groups of similar people, like the family, providing economic or psychological resources that protect against material hardship and risks of uncertainty. Strong ties can also become a basis for the pursuit of narrow interests, however, and exacerbate social divisions if homogeneous networks reinforce instead of diminish social cleavages (Molenaers 2005; Arnall et al. 2013; Dasgupta and Beard 2007; Platteau 2004; Portes 2000, 3).

24. Evidence of the impact of social capital on the effectiveness of health interventions, for instance to combat HIV/AIDS, confirms the importance of citizen engagement and community organizations (Riehman et al. 2013, 67; Campbell et al. 2013, 114; Dramé et al. 2013).

25. Tavits (2006) finds that while more civic communities in the US and Germany are more effective in demanding accountability and pressuring their local governments to deliver public goods and services, social capital does not enhance the administrative efficiency of local government organizations.

26. In response to Putnam's *Making Democracy Work*, Sidney Tarrow argues that the differential performance of Italy's subnational governments depends on the quality of political institutions in the past rather than the vibrancy of civil society (1996, 394; Skocpol, Ganz, and Munson 2000, 542).

27. As Foley and Edwards put it, "Where the state is unresponsive, its institutions are undemocratic, or its democracy is ill designed to recognize and respond to citizen demands, the character of collective action will be decidedly different than under a strong and democratic system" (1996, 48).

28. The latter example is particularly compelling as donor organizations, including the World Bank and USAID, had assessed the role of Rwandan civil society *before* the genocide as *pro-democratic* and expected it to play a major role in democratization (Armony 2004, 201). But civil-society organizations were unable to counteract the social and political forces that drove the genocide in Rwanda and were also directly involved in mass killings (Armony 2004, 201–204).

29. The study examines the determinants of grand corruption across subnational regions within European countries and tests whether formal bureaucratic institutions condition the effect of citizen-led oversight mechanisms on corruption control (Larsson and Grimes 2022). The authors find that transparent and merit-based bureaucratic governance functions as a substitute for civil-society-based accountability action, implying that civic engagement lowers corruption most in environments that lack strong institutions of bureaucratic governance.

30. Action resources widen the scope of activities that people can pursue at will and include material, intellectual, and connective resources (Welzel 2013, 18). Intellectual resources are provided by widespread education and broad access to information. Material resources are based on access to tools and equipment that ease daily life and increase productivity, leading to higher incomes. Connective resources involve access to transportation and communication technologies, facilitating exchange and coordination with others for common purposes.

31. Persson, Rothstein, and Teorell argue that monitoring public authorities and service providers will be largely ineffective if corruption is the expected behavior

because there will be no collective effort to hold corrupt officials accountable (2013). The incentives do not change even if citizens, politicians, or service providers have perfect information and even if there is broad consensus that society would be better off without corruption. The reason is that "principals cannot trust that most other actors will refrain from corrupt practices so they have no reason to refrain from paying or demanding bribes" (457). Hence the shared expectations about other actors' behavior undermine the incentives to solve the collective-action problem.

32. Cultural contexts have evolved over many centuries through the interplay of environmental factors, modes of production, philosophical and religious ideas, and formal institutions (Welzel et al. 2025; Schulz et al. 2019; Thomson et al. 2018; Talhelm et al. 2014).

33. In societies where a person is understood as independent, people tend to experience themselves as relatively autonomous from their social and physical context, free from tradition and history, and equal to others. By contrast, in societies where a person is understood as interdependent, people are more likely to experience themselves as connected and defined by relations to others, rooted in tradition and history, and embedded in existing hierarchies. Thus, in interdependent cultures, people tend to emphasize their social obligations and duties, and they pursue relational goals that align their own behavior with the needs and perspectives of in-group others (Markus 2016, 162).

34. Han's study shows that civic and political organizations play a crucial role in developing issue commitments that determine individuals' motivation for action and increase the likelihood that citizens engage in community affairs by linking their personal goals with political activities (2009).

35. Protecting the safety and security of citizens is the most basic form of governance and depends on whether the state holds the monopoly over the use of violence and defends its political sovereignty against external interference. In fragile states where governments lack the capacity to maintain social order and control military forces, independent movements, rebel groups, and warlords persistently challenge a regime through revolutionary uprisings and political violence (Norris 2012, 44–46).

36. Weber also distinguishes a charismatic type of state capacity resting on "devotion to the specific and exceptional sanctity, heroism or exemplary character of an individual person, and of the normative patterns or order revealed or ordained by him (charismatic authority)" (1947, 328).

37. Bureaucratic governance is conceptually closely related to the concept of "Quality of Government" (Rothstein and Teorell 2008), while corruption is viewed as an umbrella concept that combines the concepts of patronage, clientelism, and patrimonialism (Varraich 2014).

38. "Patronage" is defined as "the proffering of public resources (most typically, public employment) by officeholders in return for electoral support," whereas "clientelism" can be defined as "the proffering of material goods in return for electoral support" (Stokes 2013, 649–650). Even though both are conceptually related, they differ to the extent that "clientelism" implies that the more powerful political actor may or may not hold public office and, therefore, may or may not be able to credibly promise to secure public resources (such as subsidies, loans, medicines, food) for the client.

Conversely, "patronage" implies that the patron holds public office and distributes state resources (Stokes 2013, 650–651).

The concept of "patrimonialism" blends both clientelism and patronage with the difference that the focus is on the "head" of the organization. It has been mainly applied in the context of corruption in African political systems. That is, "patrimonialism" refers to the exchange of resources like jobs or licenses between high-ranking government officials and strategically located individuals (e.g., leaders of trade unions, businesspeople, or community leaders) that provide economic and political support in return (Theobald 1982, 552 cited in Varraich 2014, 21).

39. McGuire (2020) presents an excellent overview of studies on the effects of democracy on population health, focusing on the role of electoral contestation and participation (including modes of participatory governance), freedom of expression and association, long-term democratic experience, and certain democratic institutions such as parliamentarism and proportional representation. The study reveals mixed findings for electoral participation and contestation but a largely positive impact from institutionalized participatory governance mechanisms. The evidence further suggests that NGO activities, the number of political parties, proportional representation, and long-term democratic experience are positively related with population health. Conversely, labor movements and parliamentarism show little or no significant association with health outcomes. The author further reviews studies that view democracy as a moderating variable but focuses thereby mainly on research on the differential effects of economic variables (McGuire 2020, chapter 5).

40. Additionally, chapter 5 specifies bottom-up and top-down accountability mechanisms as moderators of health aid within the same model, allowing for directly comparing the impact of civic engagement vs. formal democratic oversight institutions. In other words, the analysis explores whether differences in health aid effectiveness result primarily from variations in countries' formal democratic institutions or citizens' associational involvement facilitating increased citizen participation in bottom-up processes of performance oversight.

41. Selectorate theory builds upon the assumption that political leaders attempt to stay in power and maintain control to provide either private goods to supporters or public goods, including civil liberties, to all citizens. Increasing public-good provision lowers citizens' desire for fundamental change. By contrast, decreasing the provision of public goods impedes oppositional mass movements and political coordination.

42. The reason is that the provision of public goods becomes relatively cheaper as the number of supporters increases. At the same time, receiving aid increases revolutionary threats, particularly in non-democratic, small-coalition systems where citizens benefit most from a regime change compared to the status quo.

43. Citizen demand comprises citizen actions seeking to hold providers and officials accountable, including monitoring service provision, activating horizontal oversight agencies, or engaging in elite-challenging actions. A special case of citizen-led accountability action is citizens' direct involvement in participatory development projects, which spans from design and planning to operation, maintenance, and evaluation.

3

Analyzing Conditions of Aid Effectiveness

Whether aid positively or negatively impacts development outcomes—and under which conditions—is a controversial question. Despite often relying on the same data, scholars frequently hold divergent views on the effectiveness of aid. This chapter aims to shed light on this debate. It begins by detailing the conceptualization and measurement of civic engagement, political institutions, and development assistance for health, clarifying the kind of citizen participation and political context that make aid more effective. The chapter then addresses key methodological challenges related to assessing the effectiveness of development assistance before outlining the empirical approach and the estimation strategy adopted in this study.

Measuring Civic Engagement: The Cultural Context

Some authors contend that "civic engagement" has turned into a catch-all term for almost anything that citizens might happen to do, echoing Giovanni Sartori's concerns about conceptual stretching (Berger 2009, 335). In this study, civic engagement is defined as "any activity, individual or collective, devoted to influencing the collective life of the polity" (Macedo et al. 2005, 6), encompassing nonprofessional, voluntary activities located in or targeted at the sphere of politics and actions aimed at solving collective or community problems (Van Deth 2016, 8–11). Community activities and involvement in associations with no political object are referred to as "social engagement," while activities aimed at affecting (directly or indirectly) government action are termed "political engagement" (Verba, Schlozman, and Brady 1995, 9). Within political engagement, I further differentiate between elite-challenging modes (like attending lawful demonstrations, signing petitions, or joining boycotts) and elite-entrusting modes (such as voting, contacting officials, or associating with professional interest groups). By differentiating between social and political engagement and, consequently, between community's potential and its actual demand for accountability, this study aims to refine our understanding of civic engagement and avoid its misuse as a catch-all term that has been associated with many desirable outcomes (Berger 2009).

To measure social and political engagement, I use data from various sources, including international public-opinion surveys and expert ratings. The World Values Survey (WVS) provides public-opinion data about citizen participation in more than 60 aid recipient countries from 1990 to 2014 (wave 2 to wave 6) (Inglehart et al. 2014). Additionally, the Varieties of Democracy (V-Dem) project (Coppedge et al. 2019) offers a large set of indicators that measure the vibrancy of civil society and the quality of democracy in over 100 aid recipient countries. The V-Dem indicators are based on aggregated ordinal ratings provided by country experts, with at least five experts per country and question, using Bayesian factor analysis (Pemstein et al. 2015). For more details on these data sources, refer to table A3.2 and table A3.3.

Using WVS data, we can differentiate between political engagement associated with political and professional organizations and social engagement linked to leisure and welfare organizations as well as faith-based associations.[1] Political and professional organizations—such as political parties, labor unions, and professional organizations—are usually inward-oriented, focusing on rent-seeking activities that defend their members' interests (Knack and Keefer 1997). In contrast, outward-oriented leisure and welfare organizations—such as charitable, cultural, recreational, and environmental organizations—are noted for their public-good orientation and have thus been at the center of scholarly attention among neo-Tocquevillians (Putnam 1993).[2] While faith-based associations are sometimes classified as leisure and welfare organizations, they tend to be more hierarchically organized and less connected to other voluntary associations than their nonreligious counterparts (Paxton 2007), and thus warrant separate consideration and study. To further understand the intensity of social and political engagement using WVS data, I distinguish between individuals' active (social and political) engagement, measured by the percentage of population volunteering, and passive (social and political) membership, indicated by the share of population belonging to a voluntary association.

Additional Measures of Social Engagement

To deepen the analysis of social engagement and expand coverage, I rely on two supplementary sources. First, I use the "clubs and associations" index from the Indices of Social Development database to measure a nation's aggregated level of participation in voluntary activities and voluntary time spent on unpaid community work (ISD 2013).[3] This index, hereafter referred to as Social Engagement Index (SEI), combines behavioral and perceptual indicators from public-opinion surveys with perceptual expert judgments and proxy variables (Foa and Tanner 2012, 23–27). Second, I use the CSO Participatory Environment indicator from the V-Dem project to capture the strength of civil society and its capacity to demand accountability. This index measures whether a country's citizenry is voluntarily active in a diverse set of civil-society organizations—such as labor unions, spiritual organizations (if they are engaged in civic or political activities), social movements, professional associations, charity organizations—or whether civil-society activity is mainly state sponsored (Coppedge et al. 2019, 275). Additionally, I use V-Dem data on citizens' engagement in independent nonpolitical associations. This measure, hereafter termed Non-Political Engagement, captures the share of a country's population that actively participates in sports clubs, literary societies, charities, fraternal groups, or support groups (Coppedge et al. 2020, 216).

Additional Measures of Political Engagement

To understand the role of political engagement, I distinguish between citizen involvement in elite-entrusting and elite-challenging actions. For elite-entrusting political engagement, I use different indicators from the V-Dem database that measure the share of citizens being active in political and professional associations and the extent to which civil society is capable of translating activism into political influence and holding governments accountable. These measures include the Civil Society Participation index, the Diagonal Accountability index, and two indicators of citizen involvement in political associations and trade unions, which are averaged into a Political and Professional Engagement index (detailed in table A3.3).[4]

Regarding elite-challenging actions, political engagement can aim to change government action (like improving service delivery) or seek a change of the government system (Harris and Hern 2018).[5] To capture the nuances of elite-challenging political engagement, I distinguish between elite-challenging actions related to valence issues, ideological motives, and regime change. In particular, using public-opinion data from the World Values Survey, I create an index of peaceful Social Movement Activity (SMA) based on whether individuals have participated or would participate in elite-challenging actions, such as signing a petition, joining a boycott, or attending a lawful demonstration.[6] Evidence from protest research suggests that the SMA index captures primarily peaceful accountability actions related to better service delivery (Salehyan et al. 2012).[7] To contrast this index with more ideologically oriented movements and system-changing protests, I use two additional V-Dem indicators: the Mobilization for Democracy index and the CSO Anti-System Movements index. The former measures the frequency of pro-democratic mass events such as demonstrations, strikes, and sit-ins that seek to protect or advance political rights or civil liberties (henceforth referred to as Pro-Democratic Movements) (Coppedge et al. 2020, 214). The Anti-System Movements indicator measures the extent to which peaceful or armed movements seek to change the polity in a fundamental way, thereby posing a threat to incumbent political leaders (Coppedge et al. 2019, 182). Distinguishing between pro-democratic and anti-system movements reflects differences in mass movements that seek to "change what is done by those in power" from those that seek to "change who is in power" (Harris and Hern 2018, 7). It further allows testing whether movements that can pose a real threat to political leaders undermine aid effectiveness in undemocratic recipient countries.

In sum, this study evaluates the impact of civic engagement using multiple indicators that reflect different aspects of a country's cultural context. Differentiating between social engagement, on the one hand, and elite-challenging and elite-entrusting political engagement, on the other, avoids the problem of conceptual stretching and facilitates a more precise examination of the contextual conditions that impact aid effectiveness.

Measuring Political Context

This study posits that health aid is most effective in recipient countries with both an engaged citizenry and strong formal political institutions. Essential to strengthen the impact of citizen demand for accountability is a political context characterized by a strong state, democratic institutions, and decentralization. Strong administrative capacities ensure the efficient targeting of foreign aid to populations in need. Democratic institutions provide protected spaces for citizen participation, and formal oversight mechanisms—including an independent judiciary—act as a check against governmental abuses. Decentralization allows communities to have a real say in the planning and implementation of local development interventions. The following section delves into the data used to operationalize countries' political contexts (detailed further in table A3.3). The last part outlines the measurement of other relevant determinants of public health, including socioeconomic and sociopolitical factors.

State Capacity

To measure the administrative capacity of the "Weberian bureaucracy," this study applies three widely used indicators: the Quality of Government index of the International Country Risk Guide (ICRG), the State Fragility index from the Center for Systemic Peace, and a set of indicators of corruption control from the Varieties of Democracy database.

The Quality of Government index measures levels of corruption, law and order, and bureaucracy quality, which closely mirror the Weberian distinction between legal-rational and traditional authority. The combined index captures levels of corruption in the form of excessive patronage and nepotism, the strength and impartiality of the legal system, and the capacity of the bureaucracy to deliver public services continuously without interruptions, and their autonomy from political pressure (Teorell et al. 2018, 371–372).[8]

The State Fragility index is based on the assumption that any assessment of a state's ability to win the loyalty of its people depends on its capacity to manage conflict, to make and implement public policy, and to deliver essential services—as well as its systemic resilience in responding effectively to challenges and crises and sustaining progressive development (Marshall and Elzingha-Marshall 2017, 51). The State Fragility index thus captures the effectiveness and the legitimacy of a state based on its political, economic, security, and social performance. Low state fragility implies high state capacity and strong bureaucratic governance.

The V-Dem dataset allows us to further distinguish between different forms of corruption, including public-sector corruption as well as executive, political, and regime corruption (Coppedge et al. 2019). Public-sector corruption is specified as a standard control variable and measures the extent to which public-sector employees misappropriate public resources for private use. Executive, political, and regime corruption are used to explore the interactive relationship between civic engagement and state capacity and thus to shed light on the type of corruption that conditions the effectiveness of citizen participation. While the Executive Corruption index proxies to what extent members of the executive grant favors in exchange for bribes, kickbacks, or other material inducements, the Political Corruption index summarizes corruption, bribery, and theft among members of the executive, the legislature, and the judiciary, and among public-sector employees. Additionally, I apply the Regime Corruption index, which measures how politicians use their offices for private or political gain. It focuses more specifically on corrupt behavior among high-ranking government officials who exchange resources like political office or licenses and strategically located individuals (e.g., leaders of trade unions) that provide economic and political support in return. This measure is closely linked to the concept of patrimonialism and the study of corruption in African political systems.

Democracy

To explore the interaction between civic engagement and different elements of liberal democracy, I use two frequently used comprehensive democracy indices—the Polity IV and Freedom House indices—and a set of indicators that capture the presence of specific horizontal accountability mechanisms. The Freedom House index is based on the annual Freedom in the World survey conducted by regional experts who evaluate the rights and freedoms enjoyed by individuals. Data is available for more than 190 countries from 1972 onward. The index assesses the presence of institutional checks and balances constraining the executive through the existence of a representative and inclusive legislature, an independent judiciary, and the guarantee of political rights and civil liberties, including the presence of free and fair election laws (Norris 2012, 52–53). Despite its popularity, the Freedom House index has been subject to considerable criticism due to a lack of transparency, reliability, and consistency in coding decisions and issues of concept-measure consistency (Munck and Verkuilen 2002). Specifically, the multiple dimensions included in the combined index not only assess components of minimalist definitions of democracy but also of liberal notions of democracy, including the existence of periodic, competitive elections and a broad range of political rights and civil liberties. Moreover, the equal weighting and substitutability of each item implied by their additive aggregation rule have been criticized (Munck and Verkuilen 2002, 25).

Another measure of democracy, which is widely used for monitoring regime change and studying the effects of regime authority, is provided by the Polity project initiated by Eckstein and Gurr (1975). The Polity IV project provides annual observations from 1800 to the present about the quality of democracy across the globe. The underlying concept of democracy is based on three elements: the presence of institutions and procedures through which citizens can express preferences about alternative policies and leaders, the existence of institutionalized constraints on the power of the executive, and the guarantee of civil liberties to all citizens, including political participation (Marshall, Gurr, and Jaggers 2014, 14–15). Conversely, autocracies are defined as political regimes that restrict or suppress competitive political participation, in which chief executives are selected within the political elite, and once in office, they exercise power with few institutional constraints. Against this backdrop, the Polity project scores countries' level of institutionalized democracy based on two additive scales—a democracy scale and an autocracy scale—assuming that elements of democratic and autocratic authority may coexist in any particular regime context (Marshall, Gurr, and Jaggers 2014, 17). The combined Polity score is computed by subtracting the autocracy score from the democracy score and ranges from strongly democratic (+10) to strongly autocratic (−10).[9] The Polity index has also been subject to criticism because of redundancy, conflation, and issues of concept-measure inconsistency due to the selection of an additive aggregation rule (Munck and Verkuilen 2002, 14–26). Yet, despite this criticism, the Polity IV and Freedom House index remain indicators of institutionalized democracy that are widely used in comparative politics.

While comprehensive democracy indices seek to operationalize the multidimensional concept of democracy in a single indicator, they do not allow conclusions to be drawn about the role of specific formal accountability mechanisms. Thus, further examination of the interplay between bottom-up and top-down accountability mechanisms requires using less aggregated indicators of democratic quality. For this reason, this study also applies indicators from the V-Dem project that measure the extent to which the judiciary, the legislature, and other oversight agencies hold the government accountable. In particular, I use the V-Dem indices of Legislative and Judicial

Constraints on the Executive to capture the extent of oversight by the legislature (and government agencies, such as an ombudsman or a general prosecutor) and the extent to which the executive respects the constitution and complies with court rulings (Coppedge et al. 2019). Additionally, I apply the Executive Oversight index, which focuses on oversight over the executive by government agencies only. Summarizing the extent to which the judiciary, the legislature, and other oversight agencies hold the government accountable, I also use the Horizontal Accountability index. This composite index of government accountability captures the power of state institutions to oversee the government by demanding information, questioning officials, and punishing improper behavior in order to prevent the abuse of power (Coppedge et al. 2019).

Lastly, this study applies an index that seeks to directly measure the extent to which democratic institutions shape politicians' incentives for public-good provision and has been widely used in research on comparative authoritarianism (Bueno de Mesquita and Smith 2010; Bueno de Mesquita et al. 2002). Data for index construction is taken from the Polity IV dataset (Marshall, Gurr, and Jaggers 2014) and the Cross-National Time-Series Data Archive (Banks 2015). The index combines the openness and competitiveness of executive recruitment and the party system with the independence of the legislature, and it builds upon the idea that politicians' incentives to provide public goods depend on the number of supporters a leader needs to stay in power and the size of the pool from which these supporters are drawn (Bueno de Mesquita and Smith 2010, 937; Bueno de Mesquita et al. 2002).

The number of supporters is measured by the size of the winning coalition, which is a function of the political regime. The more open and competitive the process of executive recruitment and the more competitive the country's party system, the larger the number of supporters a leader needs to stay in power. That is, the larger the size of the winning coalition. Selectorate theory predicts that as coalition size increases, it becomes more expensive for leaders to reward the rising number of coalition members through private rewards, and leaders must shift to provide more public instead of private goods (Bueno de Mesquita and Smith 2010, 937).

The size of the pool from which the supporters of a political leader can be drawn determines the ease of being replaced by others and hence supporters' loyalty to the incumbent. It is proxied by the size of the selectorate—the smaller the size of the selectorate, the lower supporters' loyalty to the incumbent. To combine leaders' support necessary to stay in power and the size of the selectorate into a composite index, I calculate the ratio of coalition size to selectorate size, which is referred to as the Coalition to Selectorate Size (CSS) ratio. Both a larger coalition size and a smaller selectorate size decrease supporters' loyalty to the incumbent and hence create incentives for political leaders to provide public goods in order to remain in office and to protect themselves against defections by members of their winning coalition (Bueno de Mesquita et al. 2003, 122). The resulting CSS ratio is strongly correlated with other democracy measures, in particular the Polity IV index ($r = 0.81$, $N = 612$, $p < 0.001$) as democratic systems tend to have larger selectorates and larger coalitions than autocratic systems.

Decentralization

Decentralization is a multidimensional process of transferring power, responsibilities, and resources from central to local authorities. It involves political, administrative, and fiscal elements and may vary in its degree of autonomy granted to the subnational units. The strongest degree of autonomy is often referred to as "devolution," which implies that local governments (1) are autonomous and perceived as separate levels of government over which central authorities exercise little or no direct control, (2) have legally recognized geographical boundaries within which they exercise authority and perform public functions, (3) have the power to secure resources to perform their functions, and (4) are perceived by local citizens as organizations providing public services that satisfy their needs and as governmental units over which they have some influence (UNDP 1997, 6–7).

Political decentralization refers to the transfer of legislative and executive power, while administrative decentralization concerns the transfer of decision-making authority and responsibility to subnational levels. As data on fiscal decentralization—meaning, subnational autonomy over expenditures and revenues—is unavailable for most countries, this study concentrates on administrative and political decentralization using data from the Database of Political Institutions (Beck et al. 2001) and the V-Dem project (Coppedge et al. 2019). Based on the former database, I use a binary indicator of administrative decentralization, which measures whether subnational governments have extensive taxing, spending, or regulatory authority.

Furthermore, I use a binary variable of political decentralization, which indicates whether the executive and the legislature at the subnational level are locally elected.

The V-Dem database provides a set of additional indicators that measure whether a regional or local government exists, and whether their executives are elected, and the extent to which locally/regionally elected offices can operate without interference from unelected bodies (i.e., their relative power). To combine the election of regional/local governments with their relative power into a composite index, I use the Regional Government and Local Government indices. Higher scores indicate that regional/local governments are elected and can operate without interference from unelected actors at the regional/local level except for the judiciary (Coppedge et al. 2020, 52).

Other Context Factors

Lastly, to answer the question of whether ordinary citizens can make aid work, it is essential to isolate the conditioning effect of civic engagement and control for alternative explanatory variables that the public-health literature has identified, including socioeconomic and sociopolitical determinants. Relevant socioeconomic determinants include a country's level of economic development, the size of the population, and whether the country is involved in violent conflicts. Including economic development as a control variable accounts for poorer countries receiving more foreign aid and having higher mortality levels (Lane and Glassman 2007, 939). To control for the level of economic development, I use log-transformed GDP per capita in constant international US\$, which is found to be negatively correlated with (log-transformed) infant mortality levels ($r = -0.8$, $N = 353$, $p < 0.001$).

The size of the population is another important determinant, as countries with larger populations may be more likely to receive foreign aid due to the higher number of people in need (Winters and Martinez 2015, 523; Acht, Mahmoud, and Thiele 2014, 25). Conversely, if donors assume economies of scale in providing health aid, they would rather allocate development assistance to countries with smaller populations, where health aid per capita has a larger effect on population health (Wilson 2011, 2039). Moreover, assuming that some donors use health aid to ensure international political support, smaller recipients are more likely to receive health aid because—regardless of size—all countries have one vote in the UN General

Assembly (Fielding 2011, 761). Hence, to control for the effects of population size, all models control for the (log-transformed) number of people living in a recipient country.

I also control for conflict involvement to account for declines in population health due to the experience of war and war-induced diseases (Krug et al. 2002, 222). The binary variable measures whether a country is involved in intrastate or interstate conflicts with more than 1,000 battle-related deaths using data from the Uppsala Conflict Data Program. Levels of infant mortality (log-scale) are found to be significantly lower (t[351] = −3.37, p < 0.001) in recipient countries not involved in conflicts (M = 3.32, SD = 0.86) compared to those involved in violent conflicts (M = 3.81, SD = 0.72).

To account for sociopolitical determinants of public health, I further control for a country's fertility rate, levels of female education, the prevalence of HIV/AIDS, the size of the health workforce, and the amount of health expenditures. Additionally, I control for public sector corruption to account for the extent to which public-sector employees misappropriate public health resources for private use (Coppedge et al. 2019).

The fertility rate captures the quality of reproductive health care and is an important determinant of population health as fewer births per woman are likely to decrease infant mortality levels by allowing parents to devote more time and resources to each child (McGuire 2010, 58–59; Dyson 2013; Murtin 2013). Simultaneously, infant mortality determines fertility because it reduces the demand for children to attain a desired number of surviving offspring as insurance for old age support or to enhance the reproduction of lineage.[10] Fertility is measured as a country's average in total births per woman (log-transformed) and is found to be strongly associated with higher levels of mortality (r = 0.84, N = 353, p < 0.001).

Socioecological approaches and behavioral health models have repeatedly emphasized the influence of education and counseling, particularly among women (Östlin, George, and Sen 2001). Specifically, female education reduces child mortality through increased use of health services (such as prenatal and postnatal care), improved maternal and child nutrition, and better access to information through empowerment and economic independence of women (Gakidou et al. 2010). Furthermore, female education influences population health by improving women's access to better working conditions. To account for female educational attainment, I use the average years of schooling among females above the age of 15. Among the sample of recipient countries, female education is negatively correlated with infant mortality ($r = -0.82$, $N = 353$, $p < 0.001$).

Furthermore, previous evidence suggests that countries with higher HIV/AIDS prevalence show increased levels of infant mortality (Mishra and Newhouse 2009, 862) and, at the same time, receive more health aid (Lane and Glassman 2007, 939). To account for the influence of the HIV disease, I control for the log-transformed prevalence of HIV/AIDS in percent of the population aged 15–49. The bivariate correlation between log-transformed HIV/AIDS prevalence and infant mortality is significantly positive ($r = 0.50$, $N = 353$, $p < 0.001$).

The scarcity of health-care workers and trained physicians is another important factor influencing population health in developing countries (Turner et al. 2016). To account for the number of available health workers, I use the log-transformed number of physicians per 1,000 people. Based on the sample of aid recipient countries, the size of the health workforce is negatively correlated with infant mortality ($r = -0.77$, $N = 353$, $p < 0.001$). Furthermore, public-health expenditures are an obvious determinant of population health in developing countries (Farag et al. 2013). Yet studies that estimate the effect of development assistance usually do not include government spending as a control variable, as government spending is endogenous to foreign aid (Wilson 2011, 2042). As donors deliver foreign aid through NGOs and multilateral organizations to bypass recipient governments with weak state institutions, however, public-health expenditures are increasingly decoupled from health aid (Acht, Mahmoud, and Thiele 2014). Therefore, this study also tests whether the effect of health aid is robust against the inclusion of public-health expenditures in percent of general government expenditures as an additional control.[11] The correlation between public-health expenditures and infant mortality is negative but comparatively small ($r = -0.23$, $N = 353$, $p < 0.001$).

Monitoring Health Aid and Population Health

Development Assistance for Health

Data on health aid commitments from international donors is taken from AidData, which combines Official Development Assistance (ODA) from OECD bilateral donors with development finance of non-OECD bilateral donors and multilateral financial institutions (AidData 2017; Tierney et al. 2011).[12] Multilateral financial institutions include regional development banks, the World Bank, and health-related funding from the Bill and Melinda Gates Foundation (BMGF) and the Global Alliance for Vaccines and Immunization (GAVI). Health-related projects covered by Aid-Data include either loans or grants in commitment form, classified by subsector and purpose of the respective activities.[13] The applied definition of health aid includes development assistance for reproductive health care, family planning, and HIV/AIDS control, and excludes humanitarian (emergency) aid. Development assistance spent on health activities is aggregated by recipient country and year.

Data on health aid is available for the period 1990–2013. To reduce business cycle fluctuations and account for the size of a recipient country, I calculate average levels of health aid per capita by country over the five subperiods: 1990–1994, 1995–1999, 2000–2004, 2005–2009, and 2010–2013. In the most recent period, aid recipient countries have received about US$6 per capita and year on average. Among those recipients with the highest median levels of per capita health aid—about US$10 per capita and year—are sub-Saharan African countries like Cape Verde, Djibouti, and Zambia; Central American countries like Nicaragua and Belize; and Asian countries such as Papua New Guinea and Bhutan. The least health aid dependent recipients are found in Eastern Europe and the MENA region.

Population Health

Overall, donors have allocated a larger share of aid to low-income and lower-middle-income countries whose health systems have limited capacity to maintain adequate service provision, contributing to poor population health (Graves, Haakenstad, and Dieleman 2015). One of the most sensitive indicators of the state of public health is a country's infant mortality rate. It is measured by the number of infant deaths per 1,000 live births and is indicative of inadequate nutrition, poor water and sanitation supply, exposure to environmental hazards, low levels of education, and poor medical and health care.

The regions with the highest infant mortality rates are sub-Saharan Africa and Asia. Yet there has been accelerating progress in reducing infant mortality worldwide. Since 1990, the global infant mortality rate across all recipient countries has more than halved, from about 66 deaths per 1,000 live births in 1990 to about 29 in 2015. To put it differently, globally, the average annual rate of decline in infant mortality increased from 2.3 percent

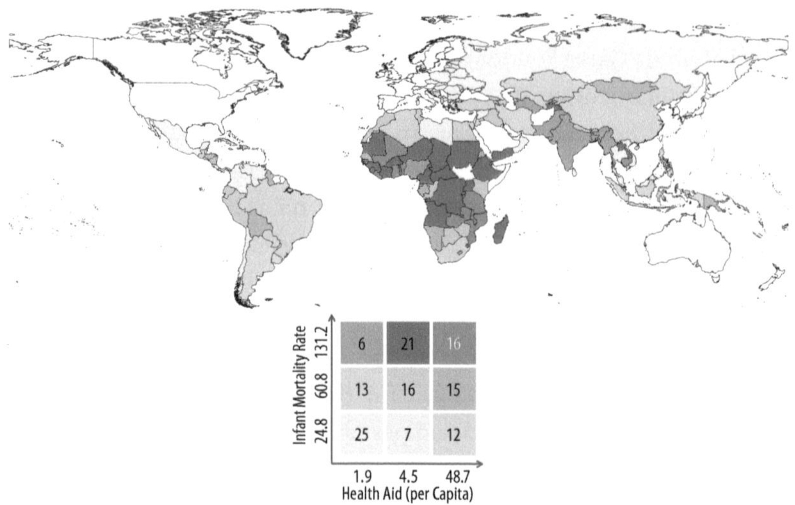

Figure 3.1. Mapping Infant Mortality and Health Aid Across Recipient Countries (1990–2015). *Note:* Shades are defined by tercile cutoffs of infant mortality rate (per 1,000 live births) and health aid per capita (in $US) averaged over the period 1990–2015. The numbers in each box of the bivariate map legend indicate the number of countries that fall within each category. Empty polygons indicate donor countries or missing data.

in 1990–1994 to 3.4 percent in 2010–2015.[14] Among those recipients with the largest declines in infant mortality are mainly Eastern European countries, including Estonia, Belarus, Georgia, the Czech Republic, and Poland. Sub-Saharan Africa, the region with the highest mortality levels in the world, has also registered a substantive acceleration. Its annual rate of decline increased from 0.6 percent in the early 1990s to 3.4 percent in 2010–2015. Annual progress has been highest in sub-Saharan African countries like Uganda, Liberia, Malawi, and Mozambique. In Asia, countries such as China, Cambodia, Bangladesh, and Nepal have experienced the highest declines in infant mortality (above 4 percent).

To visualize the distribution of health aid and the state of population health, figure 3.1 maps the average amount of health aid per capita recipient countries have obtained over the period 1990–2015 and countries' infant mortality rate. The bivariate map categorizes countries by their average levels of infant mortality and health aid over the period 1990–2015. While countries in the bottom tercile and the middle tercile received on average per capita and year up to $1.90 and $4.50 health aid, respectively, countries in the upper tercile received up to $48.70 health aid per capita and year. Within each of these categories, recipients with lower infant mortality rates (<24.8 per 1,000 live births) are shown in paler shades (desaturated), and countries with higher mortality rates (<131.2 per 1,000 live births) in darker shades (saturated).

The bivariate map clearly shows a regional clustering. Countries within sub-Saharan Africa, except Nigeria and South Africa, mainly experienced high infant mortality rates and simultaneously received medium to high levels of health aid. Conversely, Eastern Europe is characterized by low infant mortality rates and low levels of health aid dependency, except Albania and Macedonia, Bosnia and Herzegovina, and Romania and Moldova, which received higher levels of health aid. Countries within Latin America and Asia are more diverse. Within Asia, infant mortality rates vary substantially while health aid dependency is relatively modest, except in Mongolia, Nepal, Bhutan, Cambodia, Laos, and Papua New Guinea. Conversely, in Central and South American countries, infant mortality rates are generally low, but the amount of development assistance for health received varies substantially, ranging from $0.75 per capita and year in Brazil to about $9.65 in Bolivia.

It is important to mention that due to the simultaneity of the aid allocation process and the effects of health aid on infant mortality, the observed pattern between foreign aid and public health is a mix of both processes and thus must be interpreted with caution. The following section discusses this and other methodological issues in further detail and outlines how this study accounts for simultaneity bias and other sources of endogeneity.

Methodological Challenges and Solutions

In recent decades, many scholars have explored the impact of aid on developmental outcomes, using advanced analytical methods to address methodological challenges (Addison, Morrissey, and Tarp 2017; Arndt, Jones, and Tarp 2015; Stuckler, McKee, and Basu 2013). These challenges include the complexities of attributing outcomes to inputs and the fungibility of foreign aid, selection bias, and endogeneity bias caused by omitted variables, reverse causality, and measurement error. The following section delves into these challenges and their implications for this study.

Evaluating Effectiveness

Effectiveness is one of the central criteria to assess the performance of development assistance. It refers to the extent to which the development intervention's objectives are congruent with all direct effects (outcomes) resulting from the implementation of project-specific activities and the use of goods and services (outputs) (DAC 2009 26–27). Effectiveness is also used as an aggregate measure of the merit of an activity or the extent to which an intervention has attained its overarching goals, such as the MDGs.

A persistent challenge is the difficulty of attributing development outcomes solely to aid, especially given the presence of other financial flows like remittances (Bourguignon and Sundberg 2007).[15] Yet the rise of sector-wide approaches, budget support, and results-based management approaches have rendered individual donors' contributions less critical than overall progress in development outcomes. Furthermore, data on outputs of certain implementing institutions, including small NGOs, is unavailable. Thus, effectiveness studies become less concerned with the role of specific donor activities or outputs and instead focus on lasting outcomes that determine populations' health, ignoring the means for achieving the desired goals.

Another reason is that assessing the effectiveness of development interventions using output indicators can be misleading, particularly in complex areas like health-care policy. Evidence from comparative public-policy research shows that outputs, such as denser regulation, do not necessarily lead to intended outcomes and often fail to explain cross-national differences in policy outcomes (Dodds 2012, 113–120). Case-study evidence also suggests that linking donor interventions to output indicators helps little to explain the conditioning effects of institutions that are at the center of the study of political economy. In particular, Mularidharan and Sundararaman (2011) and Glewwe, Ilias, and Kremer (2010) provide evidence from randomized evaluations of teacher incentive programs in primary schools in India and Kenya, showing that teacher performance pay led to significant improvements in student test scores. But neither teacher attendance nor any other measure of teacher activity was associated with students' performance outcomes. Thus, the authors conclude that "teachers changed the effectiveness of their teaching in response to the incentives in ways that would not be easily captured even by observing the teacher" (Mularidharan and Sundararaman 2011, 69). Consequently, linking interventions to outputs (via teachers' activities) instead of students' performance outcomes may contribute little to closing the attribution gap when assessing the effectiveness of an intervention.

Moreover, the risk of incorrectly attributing health outcomes to health aid is already accounted for by governments' agreed political goals—embodied in the United Nations Millennium Declaration—which guide government action irrespective of the specific means of achieving these goals (Roller 2005, 126). Accordingly, the commitment of governments to pursue health-related MDGs already establishes the connection between external sources of health funding and health outcomes. Furthermore, studying the effectiveness of foreign aid at the macro level also allows the impact of development assistance on development outcomes to be estimated while simultaneously accounting for country-specific context conditions using econometric methods. Against this backdrop, this study focuses on the overall effectiveness of health aid and does not distinguish between specific activities implemented by different aid agencies.

Another issue in the study of aid effectiveness is the fungibility of foreign aid—that is, the diversion of aid away from its intended purpose to finance an entirely different expenditure that is usually less beneficial. For instance, recipient governments can use health aid to lower domestic taxes or to finance projects in different sectors and simultaneously reduce their own sector-specific spending. Empirical evidence on the fungibility of aid is mixed. On the one hand, Lu et al. (2010, 1382) show that for every $1 of health aid given to a recipient government, the ministry of finance reduces the amount of government expenditures allocated to the ministry of health and other government agencies that engage in health spending by about $0.43 to $1.14. These results are supported by Dieleman et al. (2013), who provide additional evidence that health aid channeled to governments is indeed fungible and "crowds out" government spending. On the other hand, Van de Sijpe (2012, 2013) only finds a limited degree of fungibility. This view is confirmed by a systematic review of evidence on the effects of aid on government spending and tax effort in recipient countries by Oliver Morrissey, who concludes that the extent to which aid is fungible is overstated. Even where it is fungible, this does not appear to make aid less effective (2015, 98).

Conversely, foreign aid may not only decrease government health expenditures (crowd-out) by freeing up domestic resources for other purposes, such as the military. Instead, aid may also increase government health spending (crowd-in), for instance aid allocated toward building health infrastructure that requires further government expenditures for additional doctors and nurses. In line with this argument, Mishra and Newhouse (2009, 870) find a positive relationship between foreign aid allocated to the health sector and government health expenditures, suggesting that health aid fosters health spending by attracting additional domestic resources allocated toward health. Against this backdrop, this study aims to test the robustness of its findings by controlling for domestic public-health expenditures (as well as non-health-related development assistance).

Endogeneity

Endogeneity is an issue that has received a lot of attention in the aid effectiveness literature. Endogeneity bias may arise from different causes, including omitted variables, reverse causality, and measurement error. Omitted variable bias occurs when a model incorrectly leaves out one or more important confounding factors (C), leading to over- or underestimation of the true effect of a predictor, such as the effect of aid on population health. Hence it is theoretically possible that health aid effectively improves population health, but we cannot observe it because we underestimate the effect size due to omitted variables. Yet this would only occur if health aid is allocated to countries that are less likely to achieve progress—for example, due to poor performance in indicators related to corruption control or state capacity.[16] On the contrary, if donors allocate aid to countries that are more likely to achieve progress, it would be less likely to underestimate health aid effectiveness.

While the aid allocation debate is ongoing, recent evidence indicates that, in the past, donors have allocated larger shares of health aid to fragile, unstable (low- and middle-income) countries to bolster their health systems and to provide long-term stability (Graves, Haakenstad, and Dieleman 2015, 1).[17] Assuming that state fragility is associated with lower population health, this allocation pattern implies that the beneficial effects of health aid are likely to be underestimated, masking health aid effectiveness.[18] This consideration is essential for interpreting the estimated effect size of health aid in cross-national studies.

Endogeneity bias also arises from reverse causality, wherein development assistance impacts population health, while simultaneously population health determines the amount of foreign aid allocated to recipient countries. In the short run, this bias can lead to a negative correlation between health aid and population health simply because poorer countries, which have higher mortality rates, are more likely to receive foreign aid (Roodman 2008; Dalgaard and Hansen 2009; Dalgaard and Hansen 2010, 39). The issue of simultaneity also applies partly to civic engagement. Citizens may become politically engaged in community activities in response to failings of public-service providers, but their engagement can also improve population health by influencing service provision and health-related agenda-setting of policymakers. Dalgaard and Hansen (2009) illustrate this so-called identification problem in the context of economic growth. Because of the simultaneity of the allocation process and the effects of foreign aid on growth, the observed correlation will always be a mix of both processes. Therefore, simple regression coefficients cannot be interpreted as reflecting a causal impact of foreign aid on development outcomes. To mitigate endogeneity concerns, this study follows an empirical approach that accounts for the potential bias induced by the simultaneity of the allocation and the effectiveness of health aid (see below).

Another source of endogeneity is measurement error, which may induce bias in the estimated regression coefficients and their standard errors and lead to incorrect significant tests and confidence intervals (Cohen et al. 2003, 119–124). The consequences of measurement error vary between outcome and predictor variables. Measurement error in outcome variables leads to increased variability of the residuals around the regression line. That is, regressing a dependent variable with measurement error on a set of explanatory factors, on average, predicts the true slope. Yet the increase in uncertainty means that confidence intervals increase in size, and the power to reject a false null hypothesis decreases (Cohen et al. 2003, 124).

Many countries, particularly those with high mortality, do not have complete information from civil registration and vital statistics systems because registering all births and deaths and recording causes of death requires considerable administrative capacity. Thus, health estimates in the poorest countries are associated with greater uncertainty levels due to a lack of reliable data (WHO 2014). Consequently, the quality of public-health data in aid recipient countries makes it harder to reject a false null hypothesis and, thus, more likely to confirm the null hypothesis that health aid is ineffective. In other words, analyzing the effectiveness of development interventions on outcomes that are measured with uncertainty makes it more likely to find insignificant effects.

By contrast, measurement error in predictor variables leads to bias in the estimated regression coefficients, resulting in regression slopes that will most likely be attenuated—meaning, be too close to zero (Cohen et al. 2003, 119). By implication, if health aid is measured with inaccuracy, its effect is likely to be underestimated, masking its effectiveness. The same applies to measures of civic engagement and formal political institutions.

Selection Bias

Despite existing studies supporting the relevance of civic engagement in the health sector, the scarcity of nationally representative data has hampered attempts to test the conditioning role of civic engagement on aid effectiveness on a comparative basis. Although recent advances in data availability allow for the analysis of larger samples of aid recipient countries, case selection remains an important issue. Selection bias can be induced by case selection on the dependent variable or by applying a selection rule that is correlated with the size of the causal effect (King, Keohane, and Verba 1995, 115–149).

A recent study on health aid effectiveness in high-mortality countries exemplifies the pitfalls of selecting on the dependent variable. The study by Wilson (2011) selects only high-mortality countries and finds no effect of health aid on mortality levels. Even though the study tests the robustness of the main findings for different levels of infant mortality (>25, >50, and >75 deaths per 1,000 life births), any of these sample selection criteria narrows the range of variation and excludes recipient countries, for example from South and Central America and Eastern Europe, that have experienced enormous improvements in population health. In other words, as the selection rule is correlated with the size of the potential effect of health aid, the reported results are likely to be underestimated.

Furthermore, in aid effectiveness studies, we observe population health only if countries receive development assistance. And, as argued above, there are good reasons to believe that the distribution of aid is not random. Thus, if we restrict our attention to aid recipients only and ignore non-aid-recipient countries, we induce selectivity bias as the unobserved factors that determine the sample selection are likely to be correlated with the dependent variable (Heckman 1979). This study follows an empirical approach that accounts for the potential selection bias induced by the nonrandom distribution of health aid, as detailed below.

Empirical Approach

This book posits that aid works better in recipient countries with both an active citizenry capable of holding governments accountable and strong political institutions, strengthening this effect. The following section lays out the empirical approach of this study to test the proposed relationships. The empirical approach is characterized by five features:

1. I test the proposed effects of civic engagement at different complementary levels of analysis. A dynamic panel study examines country-level data from aid recipients over five separate five-year periods from 1990 to 2015. A multilevel analysis study examines self-rated health among individuals and exploits variation within countries, eliminating differences linked to features of the political or socioeconomic context.

2. This study uses time lags and applies GMM estimation to mitigate the effects of simultaneity bias (Wright and Winters 2010, 66; Rajan and Subramanian 2008). Using time lags links the amount of foreign aid received in the previous period with health outcomes in the current period. Lags are also theoretically reasonable as foreign aid needs time to unfold its impact through better health infrastructure, better information, or political reform. Applying GMM estimation further mitigates the problem of reverse causality and is explained below in further detail.[19]

3. The selection rule applied in this study includes all recipient countries regardless of population health levels. The number of countries used in the analysis varies by measure of civic engagement, ranging from 52 to 101 countries (table A3.1). The V-Dem sample includes recipient countries from sub-Saharan Africa (32 percent), Latin America (21 percent), Asia (19 percent), Eastern Europe (16 percent), and the MENA region (12 percent). The WVS sample includes recipient countries from Latin America (29 percent), Eastern Europe (26 percent), Asia (18 percent), the MENA region (17 percent), and sub-Saharan Africa (11 percent). Yet, to account for the nonrandom distribution of aid, I test the robustness of the findings using dynamic Heckman two-stage selection models. To clarify, if unobserved factors that are correlated with population health determine the sample

selection and we ignore non-aid-recipient countries, we induce selectivity bias. The Heckman approach includes a first-stage probit model that captures why some countries may not receive health aid and then uses that information in the second-stage regression to compute the effect of health aid on population health (Heckman 1979).

4. This study accounts for endogeneity bias resulting from measurement errors in civic engagement and political institutions. Specifically, I apply various civic-engagement and political-context measures from public-opinion and expert surveys to mitigate the problem of measurement error. Using different measures also accounts for the issue of missing data and selection bias. Specifically, missing data is more likely in poorer, conflict-affected countries with low levels of state capacity and, consequently, is often not randomly distributed (Honaker and King 2010).

5. Besides accounting for endogeneity issues to obtain unbiased estimates of health aid, this study's primary focus is to better understand the conditions under which aid works. For this reason, I employ interaction models that test to what extent social and political engagement conditions the effectiveness of health aid and whether formal political institutions strengthen the identified effects of civic engagement (see below).

Dynamic Panel Data Estimation

In the aid effectiveness literature, GMM-type estimators, including the Arellano-Bond estimator and the Blundell-Bond-System-GMM estimator, are frequently employed to address endogeneity concerns (Baltagi 2005, 136–148).[20] Both estimators can solve the problem of endogeneity of one or more explanatory variables. The Arellano-Bond estimator applies a first difference transformation to account for country-specific (time-constant) heterogeneity and uses lagged levels of the endogenous explanatory variable as instruments for the differenced endogenous variables. The weakness of this instrumentation strategy is that the levels of endogenous regressors are often weak instruments for the first-differenced variables. Therefore, Blundell and Bond (1998) modified the Arellano-Bond estimator and included lagged levels and lagged differences into a System-GMM estimator (SYS-GMM). Exploiting these additional moment conditions improves the accuracy and efficiency of the estimates and makes SYS-GMM the preferred estimator (Baltagi 2005, 148).

Essentially, the SYS-GMM estimator predicts the effect of health aid on future population health by comparing two observably similar countries using the portion of health aid attributable to their aid histories (Mishra and Newhouse 2009, 858).[21] Simultaneously, the lagged dependent variable accounts for time-varying and time-constant historical factors that cause current differences in population health. Additionally, I include period and continent-fixed effects to control for unobserved factors that may influence population health.

It is worth noting that while GMM estimation (or instrumental variable regression in general) reduces endogeneity bias, it often results in higher standard errors. Furthermore, the application of the SYS-GMM requires that the instruments are correlated with the endogenous or predetermined regressors and satisfy the necessary orthogonality conditions—meaning, zero correlation with the error term. Additionally, SYS-GMM estimation requires no autocorrelation in the error term.[22] To check the validity of the estimations, Hansen's-J test of overidentification and a second-order serial correlation test are used.[23] A significant result (<10 percent) of the Hansen's-J test is ground to reject the joint null hypothesis that the instruments are valid (uncorrelated with the estimated error terms). In this study, Hansen's-J tests calculated from the GMM estimates are passed comfortably, supporting the validity of the generated instruments. Moreover, the results of the serial correlation test indicate the absence of second-order serial correlation, which means the estimated coefficients are not rendered inconsistent.

The dynamic panel models of this study can be estimated as a special case of the general linear model formulated in the following equation with countries indexed by i and time periods by t.

$$y_{it} = \beta_0 + \beta_1 DAH_{it} + \beta_2 CIVIC_{it} + \beta_3 DAH_{it} * CIVIC_{it} + \beta_4 X'_{it} + \beta_5 y_{it-1} + \alpha_t + \mu_i + \varepsilon_{it}$$

y_{it} measures the level of (log-transformed) infant mortality—meaning, the number of infant deaths per 1,000 live births averaged over the respective five-year period.[24] DAH_{it} reflects the amount of development assistance for health in per capita terms and $CIVIC_{it}$ refers to the extent of civic engagement, including social and political engagement, which is proposed to enhance the effectiveness of health aid. The interaction term $DAH_{it} * CIVIC_{it}$

captures the marginal effect of health aid at varying levels of civic engagement. The vector X'_{it} covers a set of control variables, including levels of GDP per capita, population size, conflict involvement and corruption control, as well as public-health expenditures, female fertility, HIV prevalence, female education, and the number of physicians. High HIV prevalence, as well as a high fertility rate, is expected to influence population health negatively. GDP per capita, public-health expenditures, control of public-sector corruption, as well as female education and the number of physicians are expected to have health-improving effects. μ_i and α_t are country-specific and period-specific fixed effects, and ε_{it} is an idiosyncratic error process.

To apply the SYS-GMM estimator, one has to distinguish between different types of regressors—exogenous, predetermined, and endogenous regressors—and specify each variable accordingly. Strictly exogenous regressors are uncorrelated with the error term and are used as instruments for themselves as in standard instrumental variable estimation. Predetermined regressors are correlated with lagged values of the error term but are uncorrelated with future errors. That is, x_{it} is a predetermined variable if the lagged error term has some feedback on subsequent realizations of x_{it} as is the case for the lagged dependent variable.[25] Endogenous explanatory variables are correlated with the contemporary errors, that is x_{it} and ε_{it} are correlated at time t.[26] For contemporaneously endogenous variables, realizations lagged by two or more periods can serve as instruments (Cameron and Trivedi 2009, 289). An endogenous explanatory variable x_{it} is thus instrumented by x_{it-2}, x_{it-3}, ... Hence, including all valid lags for endogenous variables means lags two and up.[27]

The main explanatory variables specified as endogenous include health aid, civic engagement, their interaction, and political institutions (see Chauvet 2015; Wright and Winters 2010).[28] Health aid is treated as endogenous to account for the aid allocation process, as outlined above. Civic engagement is specified as an endogenous explanatory variable because of the potential impact of participatory approaches in development assistance on community empowerment and civil-society participation through improved population health.[29] Similarly, political institutions are treated as endogenous as most authors argue that aid reduces the need for governments to be accountable to citizens and therefore undermines the quality of democracy and the quality of government.[30]

Interaction Models

Besides accounting for endogeneity issues to obtain unbiased estimates of health aid, this study's primary focus is to understand better the conditions under which aid works. For this reason, I employ interaction models that test whether and to what extent civic engagement conditions the effectiveness of health aid. Yet incorporating interaction effects is challenging and holds many pitfalls, which are frequently ignored. Reviewing the literature on multiplicative interaction models in the top-three political-science journals, Brambor, Clark, and Golder (2006, 63) demonstrate that "the execution of these models is often flawed and inferential errors are common." Additionally, Fielding and Knowles (2011) illustrate the danger of interpreting multiplicative interaction models in the context of the aid effectiveness literature. Accordingly, this subsection describes the different patterns of interactions and their interpretation to understand the effects of aid in varying cultural and political contexts.

Two predictors are said to interact with one another if the effect of each predictor on the outcome variable depends on the value of the other, which implies a combined effect on the dependent variable that is different from the sum of the effects of each individual predictor (Cohen et al. 2003, 255). Cohen et al. distinguish three theoretically meaningful patterns in two-way interactions: synergistic (enhancing) interactions, antagonistic (interference) interactions, and buffering interactions (2003, 255).[31] This distinction overlaps with the interaction relationships between formal and informal institutions proposed by Helmke and Levitsky (2004) and Lauth (2015).

A synergistic interaction pattern between health aid and civic engagement implies that both predictors affect population health in the same direction, and together they produce a stronger-than-additive effect on the outcome.[32] Given the sign of the posited relationship, a synergistic relationship is indicated if health aid is more effective in communities with high levels of civic engagement. That is, civic engagement enhances the effect of health aid (or vice versa). An antagonistic interaction pattern implies that development assistance is less important for better health in countries with high civic engagement and vice versa. To put it differently, either high levels of civic engagement or high levels of health aid improve population health. This pattern is indicated if both health aid and civic engagement work on the outcome variable in the same direction, and the interaction coefficient is of opposite sign.[33] A buffering interaction implies that one predictor weakens the effect of the other predictor on the outcome variable. In other words, as the impact of one predictor increases in value, the impact of the other predictor is diminished. This pattern is indicated if the coefficients of health aid and civic engagement are of opposite sign.[34] Correspondingly, a buffering interaction implies that civic engagement buffers the (in-)effectiveness of health aid (or vice versa).

It is essential to realize that all continuous predictors are grand mean-centered (with a mean of zero) to facilitate meaningful interpretation of interaction patterns. To clarify, mean-centering allows interpreting the first-order coefficients of health aid (X) and the moderating variable (Z) as the effects at the sample means of all other variables in the regression model. The same applies to three-way interactions with a second continuous moderator (W). Mean-centering also reduces nonessential multicollinearity between the main effect and the interaction term (Cohen et al. 2003, 267).

To facilitate interpretation, historically, interactions between continuous variables have often been analyzed by breaking the continuous variables into dichotomous categories (i.e., at the median). But dichotomization at the median involves several disadvantages: first, it strongly reduces the true association between two continuous variables, thereby lowering the power for detecting a true nonzero relationship; second, dichotomization produces spurious main effects; and third, it may also produce spurious interaction effects (Cohen et al. 2003, 256). Instead of using median split analysis, there are two alternative approaches to explore the nature of conditional relationships between two continuous variables: probing simple slopes and the Johnson-Neyman technique. Both approaches use visualizations because information about the main and interaction coefficients with the respective standard errors tells us little about the marginal effect of the explanatory variable at any observed value of the moderating variable different from zero.

Simple slope analysis involves plotting the regression of Y on X at specified values of the moderating variable (Z), typically at low, medium, and high values of Z. Even though it is common practice to specify the mean of Z, one standard deviation below the mean of Z, and one standard deviation above the mean of Z, the choice of values should be guided by the distribution of the moderating variable (Aiken and West 1991).

A more general approach is the Johnson-Neyman technique, which displays how the conditional, marginal effect of X changes across the entire range of a continuous moderating variable (Brambor, Clark, and Golder 2006; Bauer and Curran 2005). The resulting marginal effect plot provides more information than simple slope probing. In particular, it also displays the distribution of the moderating variable, which allows evaluating whether a substantial share of real-world observations falls within the range (of the moderating variable) for which the marginal effect is statistically significant.

This study applies the Johnson-Neyman technique to examine whether civic engagement makes health aid work better. To explore the interaction between the two continuous predictors, I visualize the estimated marginal effect of health aid across observed levels of civic engagement. Thus, the marginal effect plots indicate how the marginal effect of health aid changes as a country's level of civic engagement varies. At a specific level of civic engagement, health aid has a statistically significant effect on population health whenever the upper and lower bounds of the two-tailed 95 percent confidence intervals are either above or below the zero line. The overlaid histogram shows the frequency distribution of the moderating variable and guarantees that the estimated effects fall within the observed range of the sample data.

To further explore whether political-context conditions strengthen the identified moderating effect of civic engagement, I combine the Johnson-Neyman technique with post hoc probing. Specifically, to examine the interaction between the two continuous predictors and another (continuous or binary) moderator, I compare the combined effects of civic engagement and health aid at low, moderate, and high levels of institutional quality. This implies drawing the estimated marginal effect of health aid across observed levels of civic engagement for each group of countries separately. The sample mean indicates moderate levels of institutional quality. Low and high levels of institutional quality are indicated by one standard deviation below or above the sample mean. A significant three-way interaction coefficient implies that the slopes of the three marginal effect lines vary substantially and suggests that the moderating effect of civic engagement varies between countries of different institutional quality.

NOTES

1. Data from the WVS on membership in voluntary organizations is available for Wave 3 (1995–1998), Wave 5 (2005–2009), and Wave 6 (2010–2014). Leisure and welfare

organizations include associations that serve various purposes, such as sports or recreation; art, music, or education; environmentalism; and charity or humanitarianism. Political and professional organizations include political parties, labor unions, and professional organizations.

2. Putnam attributes the trust- and cooperation-enhancing function of associations to formal horizontal networks—excluding vertical networks that consist of actors of different status and power because they involve less-reliable information-sharing mechanisms and limited opportunities to sanction opportunistic behavior of the more powerful (Putnam 1993, 175). The related literature on civil society, however, has repeatedly pointed to the importance of broadening the focus beyond formally organized (horizontal) associations and distinguishing between different types and functions of social capital, including elite-challenging forms of civic engagement and more informal communal networks (Krishna 2002; Edwards and Foley 2001; Welzel, Inglehart, and Deutsch 2005; Anheier and Kendall 2002).

Anheier and Kendall suggest studying social capital within the wider context of civil society, as both concepts are closely related (2002, 355). Specifically, civil society comprises those organizations that complement states and markets, while at a lower unit of analysis, social capital involves the norms and networks of civil-society organizations that enable people to cooperate (Woolcock 2011, 197). A comprehensive discussion of the concept of civil society and its limitations can be found in the works by Alison van Rooy (2013) and Michael Edwards (2020).

3. The Social Engagement Index (SEI) covers a larger cross section of aid recipient countries and is available for the period 1990–2015 (table A3.1). The composite SEI and the WVS indicators of social engagement (belonging and volunteering) in leisure and welfare, and faith-based organizations are highly correlated. Both Cronbach's alpha (alpha = 0.87) and Raykov's reliability coefficient (Xi = 0.88) indicate high internal consistency among the different indicators of social engagement.

4. The Civil Society Participation index assesses a country's participatory environment and combines it with information about citizens' involvement in civil-society organizations, the candidate nomination process within party organizations, and women's participation in civil society. This index considers the extent to which civil-society organizations are capable of translating their activism into political influence and accounts for the presence of traditional status barriers to civil-society participation (Bernhard et al. 2017, 347). The Diagonal Accountability index measures to what extent governments are held accountable by civil-society organizations and citizen-led accountability actions, including investigative journalism and social mobilization. Lastly, I create a composite index by averaging citizens' engagement in political associations and trade unions to directly measure the share of the population active in political and professional associations. The resulting Political and Professional Engagement index captures the share of citizens being active in civil-society organizations such as environmental associations, animal-rights groups, business associations, and trade unions.

5. Harris and Hern demonstrate that service delivery is a major issue of protest events in African countries (2018). Specifically, valence protests are an expression of citizens exercising voice and demanding accountability from governing officials,

particularly in regimes where formal avenues of political engagement are insufficient for communicating preferences to the government. Thus, protests that seek to resolve a grievance over a specific valence issue are different from more ideologically oriented and system-changing protests (Harris and Hern 2018, 11).

6. The SMA index is available for Wave 2 (1990–1994) to Wave 6 (2010–2014) of the WVS, and its construction is based on the methodology suggested by Welzel (2013, 224). The index is calculated by recoding respondents' answers about whether they did do the activity, they might do it, or they would never do it. Respondents who answer "might do," indicating "readiness to act," are considered in between respondents who refuse to participate and those who have participated. Though, to give "readiness to act" less weight than action, answers are weighted down. Accordingly, "would never do it" is coded 0, "might do it" 0.33, and "have done it" 1.0. Averaging each respondent's scores over the three activities and calculating each country's population average per wave leads to the SMA index.

7. Data from the Social Conflict Analysis Database (SCAD) about protests in Africa and Central America suggests that health-service delivery is a major issue of protests in many recipient countries (Salehyan et al. 2012). In each aid recipient country for which data is available, there have been several protest events related to water and sanitation each year (between one and eleven events per year). About one-third of the events related to poor service delivery were attended by up to 10,000 participants.

8. Since the Quality of Government index has a comparatively small country coverage, I also use the Control of Corruption index from the World Bank's Worldwide Governance Indicators (WBGI) database for robustness checks (Kaufmann, Kraay, and Mastruzzi 2011). The WBGI index of corruption control measures the perceived extent to which public power is exercised for private gain as well as "capture" of the state by elites and private interests. Even though the WBGI dataset has a broader country coverage than the ICRG dataset, it also has a smaller time coverage.

9. The democracy indicator is derived from codings of the competitiveness of political participation (+1, +3), the openness (+1) and competitiveness (+1, +2) of executive recruitment, and constraints on the chief executive (+1, +4). The autocracy indicator is derived from codings of the regulation (−1, −2) and competitiveness (−1, −2) of political participation, the openness (−1) and competitiveness (−2) of executive recruitment, and constraints on the chief executive (−1, −3). To apply the index to panel data analysis, I use a modified version of the Polity variable, which converts periods of foreign "interruption," "interregnum" (anarchy), or "transition" to conventional polity scores according to the following rules: cases of foreign "interruption" are treated as missing values; cases of "interregnum" (or anarchy) are converted to a "neutral" score of 0; and cases of "transition" are prorated across the span of the transition (Marshall, Gurr, and Jaggers 2014, 17).

10. For a recent review of the empirical evidence on the causal relationship between infant mortality and fertility, see Roodman (2014).

11. Based on the classification scheme for National Health Accounts (NHA) of the World Health Organization, public-health expenditures include tax-funded health expenditures, social security for health, and external resources (including loans and grants) for medical care and medical goods channeled through a ministry of health or other public agencies (on-budget health aid). Grants to NGOs, which are not channeled

to the government (off-budget health aid), are accounted as private health expenditures (Poullier, Hernandez, and Kawabata 2002, 5–6). Private health expenditures also integrate health insurance, mandated enterprise health expenditures, and out-of-pocket expenditures in health goods. Public and private health expenditures sum up to a country's total health expenditures.

12. AidData 3.1 is available at https://www.aiddata.org/datasets, accessed on February 06, 2020.

13. Health aid activities enable governments to train health personnel, invest in buildings and equipment, and purchase health services that provide equitable access to medical products, vaccines, and safe technologies. Health aid also aims to develop administrative and management capacities that enable staff to raise and allocate funds, ensure accountability, and monitor the quality of services delivered by health-care providers. These contributions include grants and concessionary loans, provided with no interest or at a rate significantly lower than the current market rate. This definition expands the definition of Official Development Assistance (ODA) used by the OECD's Development Assistance Committee (DAC). It includes loans at market rates if governments or intergovernmental organizations extend these loans to foster socioeconomic development but excludes private flows and military assistance (Tierney et al. 2011). The DAC defines Official Development Assistance as those grants or loans to countries and territories (on the DAC List of ODA Recipients) and to multilateral development institutions that are (1) provided by the official sector, (2) administered with the promotion of the economic development and welfare of developing countries as their main objective, (3) concessional in character and—if a loan—convey a grant element of at least 25 percent (DAC 2008).

14. The average annual rate of decline in infant mortality is calculated as the difference between the current level of log-transformed infant mortality and the previous level of log-transformed infant mortality divided by the number of periods (T) between both points in time: $\frac{log(IMR_t) - log(IMR_{t-1})}{T}$.

15. Remittances from international migration provide an important flow to developing countries, which were more than three times the size of ODA in the year 2015 (World Bank 2015). Yet Chauvet, Gubert, and Mesplé-Somps (2013) demonstrate that the positive relationship between health aid and population health is robust to controlling for the amount of remittances. Furthermore, earlier studies on the health effects of aid have analyzed data on total development assistance (Gomanee et al. 2005; Masud and Yontcheva 2005), making it more difficult to establish a robust link between health outcomes and certain interventions.

16. In particular, this would only apply if aid is positively correlated with the unobserved factor C, which in turn is negatively associated with population health or vice versa. We would thus underestimate the positive effect of health aid on population health whenever the correlation of the unobserved factor with health aid is of opposite sign than its relationship with population health (Wooldridge 2013, 90).

17. Whether state institutions determine the amount of foreign aid received by developing countries remains disputed. Evidence from the aid allocation literature is ambiguous. On the one hand, those that find no association between the quality of

bureaucratic governance and the amount of foreign allocated to recipient countries argue that donors face the problem that those countries most in need typically also lack proper institutions as well as the fact that donors pursue their own interests, including commercial, conflict-mitigating and democracy-promoting purposes when giving aid (Bueno de Mesquita and Smith 2009; Hoeffler and Outram 2011; Easterly 2007). On the other hand, there is evidence that recipients with stronger state institutions receive *more* aid than their counterparts (Winters and Martinez 2015; Acht, Mahmoud, and Thiele 2014). Donors' aid allocation patterns in the health sector appear to differ, however. In particular, Graves, Haakenstad, and Dieleman (2015) demonstrate that among low- and middle-income countries, those classified as fragile because of high concentrations of armed conflict, ethnic violence, inequality, debt, and corruption received more health aid in per capita terms.

18. Specifically, assuming that state fragility is associated with lower population health, this finding implies the resulting omitted variable bias on average induces a downward biased (positive) coefficient of health aid on population health. Consequently, given that donors have allocated larger shares of health aid to fragile states, the estimated coefficient of health aid is likely to be too low and thus mask rather than overestimate the effectiveness of health aid.

19. Additionally, I include period and continent-fixed effects to control for unobserved factors that may influence population health. Moreover, dynamic panel models include the lagged dependent variable as an additional predictor, which simultaneously accounts for time-varying and time-constant historical factors that cause current differences in population health.

20. While standard panel data techniques, including error component models, are typically applied to account for time-constant unobserved factors, they do not solve the problem of time-varying omitted variables (Welzel, Inglehart, and Kruse 2017). By contrast, dynamic panel models use a lagged dependent variable to account for time-varying and time-constant historical factors that cause current differences in population health that are difficult to account for in other ways (Wooldridge 2013, 120–121, 313). Moreover, in contrast to static panel data models, which imply that the effect of aid on mortality is felt only immediately and completely within one period, dynamic panel models allow the effects of health aid to vary over time. For instance, an initial effect may increase to some limit over time, which is likely given the nature of health aid projects (Beck and Katz 2011).

21. For the SYS-GMM, two different IV-estimators can be obtained: the 2SLS estimator (two-stage-least-square), called the "one-step estimator," and the two-step estimator, which is more efficient by using optimal generalized method of moments. Since the two-step estimator shows standard errors that tend to be biased downward, Windmeijer bias-corrected robust standard errors are used.

22. More specifically, if the idiosyncratic errors are independent and identically distributed (i.i.d.), the first-differenced errors are first-order serially correlated; however, serial correlation in the first-differenced errors at an order higher than one implies valid moment conditions (Roodman 2009).

23. The Sargan and Hansen tests permit testing the exogeneity of the instruments used as long as the number of instruments is higher than the number of endogenous and

predetermined regressors (overidentification) and the error regarding the instruments is homoscedastic (Auer and Rottmann 2011, 569). The Sargan test statistic has the null hypothesis that the instruments are not correlated with the error term and are, therefore, validly excluded from 2SLS estimation. If the null is not rejected, the instruments are assumed to be valid. But if heteroscedastic (nonspherical) errors are suspected, as in the case of robust one-step GMM, the chi-squared statistics of the Sargan test are inconsistent, and the Hansen test from a two-step estimate is theoretically superior (Roodman 2009, 97–98).

Sargan's statistic is a special case of Hansen's-J under the assumption of homoscedasticity. Whether to rely on Hansen's-J or Sargan's test of overidentifying restrictions depends on whether nonsphericity in the errors (e.g., in the case of heteroscedastic errors) is suspected. For robust GMM, the Sargan test statistic is inconsistent. Nonetheless, as both tests have low power if the number of excluded instruments is high, the "Difference-in-Sargan tests of exogeneity of instrument subsets" are used as additional evidence of instrument validity.

24. Data is taken from the World Development Indicators. Applying log transformation to mortality levels reduces skewness, facilitates interpretation, and allows for a given increase in health aid to have a larger impact on mortality when the initial mortality ratio is higher (Mishra and Newhouse 2009, 857).

25. In other words, $E(x_{it}\varepsilon_{is}) \neq 0$ for $s < t$ and $E(x_{it}\varepsilon_{is}) = 0$ for $s \geq t$. To account for the absent exogeneity, a predetermined variable x_{it} is instrumented by $x_{it-1}, y_{it-2}, \ldots$ and so on. Thus, the lagged dependent variable y_{t-1}, which is predetermined, is instrumented with $y_{t-2}, y_{t-3}, \ldots$. In a dynamic panel with five periods for the LDV at t=5, there are three available instruments: $y_{i3}, y_{i2},$ and y_{i1}. At t=4 there are two available instruments: y_{i2} and y_{i1}. At t=3 there is one available instrument: y_{i1}. So the number instruments used for the LDV regressor is 3+2+1=6. The total number of instruments is the sum of the used instruments over all predetermined and endogenous regressors.

26. $E(x_{it}\varepsilon_{is}) \neq 0$ for $s \leq t$ and $E(x_{it}\varepsilon_{is}) = 0$ for $s > t$.

27. The number of instruments increases with the number of available periods, however. Too many instruments may negatively influence the robustness of the Sargan/Hansen-test statistic as well as the asymptotic properties of the estimator. Therefore, different model specifications are tested, whereby either the lag ranges used in generating the instrument sets are limited, or instruments are collapsed (Roodman 2009, 107).

28. Furthermore, depending on the model specification, additional explanatory variables that are typically treated as outcome variables in aid effectiveness studies are specified as endogenous, including all socioeconomic and sociopolitical controls.

29. Donors have channeled more official aid to and through NGOs, which may have increased the number of civil-society organizations (CSOs) that deliver social services. Thus, respondents in countries that receive large amounts of aid may be more likely to be members of CSOs and, therefore, create a positive correlation between the size of civil society and health aid. By contrast, Bano (2012) reports that development assistance is likely to decrease levels of social engagement as receiving aid funding can raise concerns about the independence of community associations from foreign influence and thus negatively affect membership. Empirically, health aid per capita is

uncorrelated with current membership in any voluntary organization, participation in elite-challenging action, and the Social Engagement Index. Only the CSO Participatory Environment index and the Civil Society Participation index show a small positive correlation with health aid of $r = 0.16$. Nevertheless, whether civic engagement is specified as an endogenous or exogenous predictor in the GMM estimation leads to qualitatively similar results.

30. For a detailed discussion on the link between aid and accountability, see chapter 2. Theoretically, political institutions can be treated as endogenous or exogenous to aid. Empirically, however, modifications of this kind lead to similar conclusions.

31. In the context of multiple regression analysis, two-way interaction models include three predictors: the two main effects (X and Z) and the interaction effect (X*Z). According to standard notation, β_1 and β_2 refer to the "main" effects, while β_3 refers to the coefficient of the interaction term. Three-way interaction models include seven predictors: the "main" effects of X, Z, and W, the two-way interaction coefficient X*Z, X*W, W*Z, and the three-way interaction coefficient (X*Z*W). Main effects are also called "first-order coefficients," while second-order coefficients refer to two-way effects, and so on.

32. A synergistic interaction pattern is indicated if all three regression coefficients show the same sign (either positive or negative): ($\beta_1 < 0$, $\beta_2 < 0$, and $\beta_3 < 0$) or ($\beta_1 > 0$, $\beta_2 > 0$ and $\beta_3 > 0$).

33. An antagonistic interaction pattern is indicated if ($\beta_1 < 0$, $\beta_2 < 0$, and $\beta_3 > 0$) or ($\beta_1 > 0$, $\beta_2 > 0$ and $\beta_3 < 0$).

34. A buffering interaction pattern is indicated if ($\beta_1 < 0$ and $\beta_2 < 0$) or ($\beta_1 < 0$ and $\beta_2 < 0$).

4

Mapping Differences in Civic Engagement Among Aid Recipient Countries

A vibrant voluntary sector is essential for an engaged citizenry to stimulate public debate and press governments for action on public matters. Evidence from several regional and country case studies supports this relationship (Almond and Verba 1963; Verba, Nie, and Kim 1971; Verba and Nie 1972; Seligson 1980; Booth and Richard 1998; Bratton, Mattes, and Gyimah-Boadi 2004; Klesner 2007, 2009). Expanding this research, this chapter probes the linkages between social and political engagement and communities' willingness and capacity to demand accountability for a large cross-section of countries. It assesses whether citizen engagement in recipient countries is infused with civic attitudes, liberal values, and cooperative norms and whether such engagement corresponds with increased participation in elite-challenging action. While the chapter establishes the link between civic engagement and bottom-up demands for accountability in recipient countries, the findings hold significant implications for donors seeking to strengthen the motivation and capacity of civil society to check the abuse of power.

The chapter proceeds as follows. The first part describes differences in social and political engagement across aid recipient countries. Second, the chapter examines to what extent social and political engagement in recipient countries is associated with political interest, support for liberal democracy, civic value orientations, and out-group trust. Moreover, it outlines the link between social engagement and citizen's participation in elite-challenging action. Against this backdrop, the third part shows how health aid and population health have coevolved over time within countries of different levels of civic engagement. Taken together, this chapter provides evidence that social and political engagement qualifies as a key moderating factor likely to influence the effectiveness of development assistance.

Social and Political Engagement in Recipient Countries

The book posits that differences in aid effectiveness are shaped by variations in citizen demand for accountability, resulting from varying levels of social and political engagement. Variation in citizen engagement is deeply rooted in a region's distinct cultural and historical context. Using data from the World Values Survey (1990–2014), table 4.1 illustrates the large variation in social and political engagement between and within world regions. Sub-Saharan Africa exhibits the highest levels of citizen engagement. Eastern Europe and the MENA region maintain the lowest levels of engagement. Furthermore, democratic societies have higher average levels of citizen engagement than authoritarian regimes.

A closer look at sub-Saharan Africa, especially East African countries like Kenya, Malawi, Ethiopia, Uganda, and Tanzania, reveals that the region's strong social engagement is largely influenced by religion. About 83 percent of the population in sub-Saharan African countries belong to faith-based organizations, and nearly half participate in leisure and welfare organizations.[1] The historical roots of civil-society organizations in Africa date back to precolonial traditions of communalism and voluntarism. In countries like Kenya and Uganda, self-help groups based on family or clan ties have been vital in promoting local welfare and mobilizing political support after the countries' independence (Kanyinga 2010, 248). Furthermore, civil-society organizations spurred democratic transition and complemented governments in the delivery of public services. In Central and Southern Africa, associational life emerged from liberation movements against colonial rule, aligning closely with oppositional parties supporting democratic transition, as seen in Zambia, Zimbabwe, and South Africa (Yachkaschi 2010, 230). Women- and human-rights organizations in this region, particularly in the Central African Republic, the Democratic Republic of the Congo, Rwanda, and Burundi, have been instrumental in peace building and humanitarian relief.

Social movements have proliferated across Africa since the late 1990s, advocating for diverse issues such as an alternative development agenda, food security, debt relief, environmental issues, land rights, women's rights, access to antiretroviral drugs, LGBTQ+ rights, and opposition to the privatization

Table 4.1. Social and Political Engagement by Country

		Social Engagement		Political Engagement	
	Any Association	Leisure and Welfare Associations	Faith-Based Associations	Political and Professional Associations	Elite-Challenging Action
Eastern Europe (EEU)	**40.4**	**18.5**	**17.4**	**24.2**	**23.6**
Albania	66.2	18.5	21.1	42.5	28.8
Armenia	58.1	52.8	49.5	55.5	24.9
Azerbaijan	35.1	10.4	3.7	27.4	15.4
Belarus	54.7	12.3	9.1	45.4	20.7
Bulgaria	20.8	6.6	3.7	14.9	14.8
Croatia	80.0	36.2	54.7	37.8	44.6
Czech Republic	53.8	30.1	16.6	26.5	26.3
Estonia	42.2	25.1	12.9	17.3	25.5
Georgia	18.0	4.9	10.0	5.1	24.9
Hungary	34.2	13.7	15.4	15.2	22.9
Kazakhstan	27.3	16.9	8.7	15.9	8.4
Kyrgyzstan	53.1	40.4	19.2	35.1	17.3
Latvia	44.0	18.8	13.4	24.5	39.1
Lithuania	32.0	13.7	13.8	12.1	34.3
Macedonia	47.1	29.9	17.7	32.8	27.0
Moldova	62.1	23.4	32.6	33.1	23.2
Poland	29.7	20.3	24.4	14.5	29.3
Romania	36.2	11.2	22.5	17.9	18.5
Russia	35.5	12.9	7.6	25.1	27.9
Slovakia	59.0	27.4	28.6	28.6	26.8
Ukraine	40.5	13.0	12.8	26.2	20.8
Uzbekistan	17.7	15.0	4.2	4.2	0.0
Middle East and North Africa (MENA)	**24.3**	**16.0**	**8.2**	**11.9**	**16.6**
Algeria	22.2	16.7	8.3	5.6	26.0
Egypt	9.2	3.8	1.2	6.6	19.0
Iran	60.7	44.7	38.9	19.6	0.0
Iraq	23.4	15.7	10.0	6.8	16.9
Jordan	15.7	9.7	6.9	5.7	8.5
Lebanon	55.5	43.8	22.2	32.7	23.1
Libya	35.1	28.9	10.0	17.1	34.5
Morocco	22.7	15.3	4.1	10.6	18.0
Tunisia	10.0	7.5	1.6	3.8	14.4
Turkey	18.4	9.6	2.7	12.1	16.7
Yemen	30.6	12.9	8.2	23.3	19.7
Sub-Saharan Africa (SSA)	**90.7**	**53.6**	**83.0**	**49.7**	**25.4**
Burkina Faso	59.9	25.2	48.7	24.7	24.0
Ghana	96.3	51.6	93.2	54.5	10.0
Mali	81.8	63.1	67.0	53.5	29.5

| | | Social Engagement | | Political Engagement | |
	Any Association	Leisure and Welfare Associations	Faith-Based Associations	Political and Professional Associations	Elite-Challenging Action
Nigeria	95.7	58.9	90.3	45.3	32.3
Rwanda	92.4	57.9	77.4	56.7	14.5
South Africa	91.1	52.9	84.3	50.7	30.6
Tanzania					35.6
Uganda					30.5
Zambia	97.8	63.8	96.0	52.0	27.3
Zimbabwe	97.1	49.3	93.0	50.6	15.0
Asia	**52.9**	**37.2**	**33.6**	**32.0**	**15.7**
Bangladesh	60.3	37.6	33.6	31.5	24.4
China	33.4	19.7	7.6	21.0	2.9
India	73.3	62.5	51.3	59.5	33.9
Indonesia	82.8	63.0	67.0	37.5	15.6
Malaysia	49.3	30.0	30.1	27.3	6.7
Pakistan	28.6	16.7	16.0	13.5	14.5
Philippines	58.4	38.3	40.8	25.9	16.6
Thailand	45.5	34.0	32.8	25.5	11.7
Vietnam	49.2	26.9	11.6	31.3	7.0
Latin America Caribbean (LACAR)	**66.0**	**37.2**	**51.3**	**22.4**	**30.8**
Argentina	52.8	31.0	36.6	17.5	30.2
Brazil	83.7	33.0	74.6	25.5	54.8
Chile	64.0	42.7	46.9	21.7	29.4
Colombia	60.3	29.5	45.8	16.6	28.3
Dominican Republic	90.9	61.5	74.0	53.1	32.9
Ecuador	46.8	20.9	35.9	10.8	15.2
El Salvador	68.1	29.2	56.4	9.6	20.5
Guatemala					14.1
Mexico	81.8	50.8	68.4	33.9	30.2
Peru	65.0	37.7	47.0	19.5	30.0
Trinidad and Tobago	82.0	44.9	76.2	28.6	29.0
Uruguay	48.5	27.7	28.7	16.2	34.4
Venezuela	62.1	40.4	44.8	25.6	24.0
Autocracies	**46.8**	**27.0**	**28.9**	**26.1**	**18.6**
Democracies	**55.1**	**31.1**	**37.8**	**26.2**	**26.3**

Note: Table reports the share of respondents being a member of (belonging to) political and professional associations, leisure and welfare associations, and faith-based associations, as well as the percentage of respondents having participated in non-institutionalized modes of elite-challenging action. Values are averaged over the period 1995–2014 based on WVS Waves 1995–1998, 2005–2009, and 2010–2014.

of public goods (Yachkaschi 2010, 233). In this context, trade unions play a pivotal role in mobilizing political action to address the pressing concerns of the vast majority living in poverty across the continent (Kew and Oshikoya 2014, 17).

Moreover, African protesters challenge not only national elites but also international financial institutions like the World Bank and the prescribed reforms that recipient countries are supposed to implement in return for funding (Yachkaschi 2010, 234). Resistance against structural adjustment policies has been most prominent in Zimbabwe, South Africa, and Zambia. Here, in 2004, trade unions mobilized large protests against the International Monetary Fund. But African civil-society organizations are often subject to repressive legislation that undermines their autonomy and puts them at risk of being coopted through patronage ties (Kew and Oshikoya 2014, 17). In particular, organizations promoting human rights and democracy must fear state repression, unlike associations engaged in service delivery that are often subcontracted by the government (Yachkaschi 2010, 233).

Civil society in the Middle East and North Africa—the region with the lowest levels of citizen engagement—is often described as ineffective, undemocratic, elitist, and dominated by patronage relations (Saber 2010, 310). In countries like Tunisia, Jordan, Algeria, and Morocco, the freedom of voluntary associations is strongly curtailed by the state, either directly through legal and administrative rules or indirectly by providing government funds to monitor activities and control civil-society organizations, including religious associations (Liverani 2010, 272). Only a minor share of the officially registered voluntary associations is active, resulting in an associational life that tends to be family or close-knit group-centered (Liverani 2010, 269). Despite the limited space for civil-society organizations, the region witnessed a significant surge in activism during the Arab Spring. This seeming paradox can be best understood by considering the role of social networks, Islam, and people's long experience of oppression and autocratic rule. Many protesters during the Arab Spring were motivated by the search for social and economic justice and a suppressed desire for political freedoms. Evidence suggests this motivation is linked to religious beliefs (rather than attendance of religious services), making citizens more sensitive to injustice and contributing to their willingness to participate in protests (Hoffman and Jamal 2014).[2] Information and communication technology, especially social-media networks, provided the means to allow dissatisfied citizens, particularly urban youth, to spread relevant information and mobilize collective actions (Ardic 2012).

For Eastern Europe, the low level of associational involvement is considered one of the enduring legacies of post-communist rule (Howard 2003).[3] For instance, in Russia, civil society has been historically shaped by the country's ruling political regime, eliminating and replacing independent associations with state-oriented organizations (Gilbert 2010). Even though under glasnost and perestroika in the 1980s, the number of associations independent of state control gradually increased, citizens' participation in voluntary associations is low by international standards. According to the New Russia Barometer in 2007, 95 percent of respondents reported not being a member of either a sports, arts, community, or charitable association (Gilbert 2010, 275). According to the World Values Survey (WVS), only about 13 percent of the Russian population is a member of a leisure and welfare association.

In Asia, social engagement is moderately high by international standards, while political engagement is particularly low in China, Malaysia, and Vietnam. Associational involvement is highest in South and Southeast Asia and is dominated by faith-based organizations. Specifically, in countries such as Bangladesh, Malaysia, Thailand, and the Philippines, about one-third of the population is a member of a faith-based organization. Similarly, on average, more than 50 percent of the Asian population report regularly spending time once or more a week at a church, mosque, or temple to socialize (Weiss 2010, 296). Likewise, development-oriented, educational, and humanitarian organizations have expanded in the whole region. For instance, India has many politically oriented organizations rooted in its long history of nationalist movements and high levels of political engagement (Blomkvist and Uba 2010, 292). In countries such as Indonesia and the Philippines, where governments exercise less control over civil society, trade unions and NGOs play an essential role in public life (Weiss 2010, 298; Alagappa 2004). Even in more repressive environments like Vietnam, community welfare organizations and business associations provide an important resource for mobilizing political action (Weiss 2010, 297).

Latin America and the Caribbean is the region with the second-largest level of social engagement and the largest level of political engagement. The region has a long tradition of faith-based organizations complementing governments in delivering public services (Roitter 2010). On average, about half of the Latin American population is a member of a religious organization. After the transition toward consolidated democracies in the mid-1990s, emerging advocacy and empowerment-based organizations complemented existing elite-oriented educational and faith-based organizations. Since then, the number of voluntary associations and their contribution to the provision of public services has increased. In Central America, civil society was politicized under military dictatorships at the end of the 20th century, as in Guatemala, El Salvador, and Nicaragua. Similarly, civil-society organizations played a crucial role in transitioning toward democracy, particularly by monitoring elections and promoting citizen participation (Natal, Cadena-Roa, and Rappoport 2010, 264). Civil-society organizations in Latin America continuously touch upon redistribution, environmental problems, and Indigenous rights.

Besides these cross-national differences, it is vital to examine to what extent civic engagement in aid recipient countries varies over time. Figure 4.1 displays the variation in social and political engagement within countries from 1990–2015 based on expert ratings from the V-Dem project. The more extensive longitudinal coverage of the V-Dem data allows for examining the temporal variation in civic engagement in further detail. The reported violin plots visualize each country's median level and interquartile distribution of the share of the population that actively participates in independent non-political associations as well as in political associations and trade unions (figure 4.1).

The reported evidence suggests that for most aid recipient countries, social and political engagement levels vary little over time. In some countries, however, substantial transformations have affected levels of social and political engagement, yet to a different extent. The pooled country-level

---

Figure 4.1. *(opposite)* **Within-Country Variation in Social and Political Engagement (1990–2015).** *Note:* The figure shows the variation of social and political engagement within countries over the period 1990–2015. Each violin plot displays a country's median (circled marker), interquartile range (black box), and estimated kernel density. Social engagement is measured using V-Dem's Non-Political Engagement index, which measures the share of the population that actively participates in independent non-political associations. Political engagement is measured using the Political and Professional Engagement index, which captures citizens' participation in political associations and trade unions.

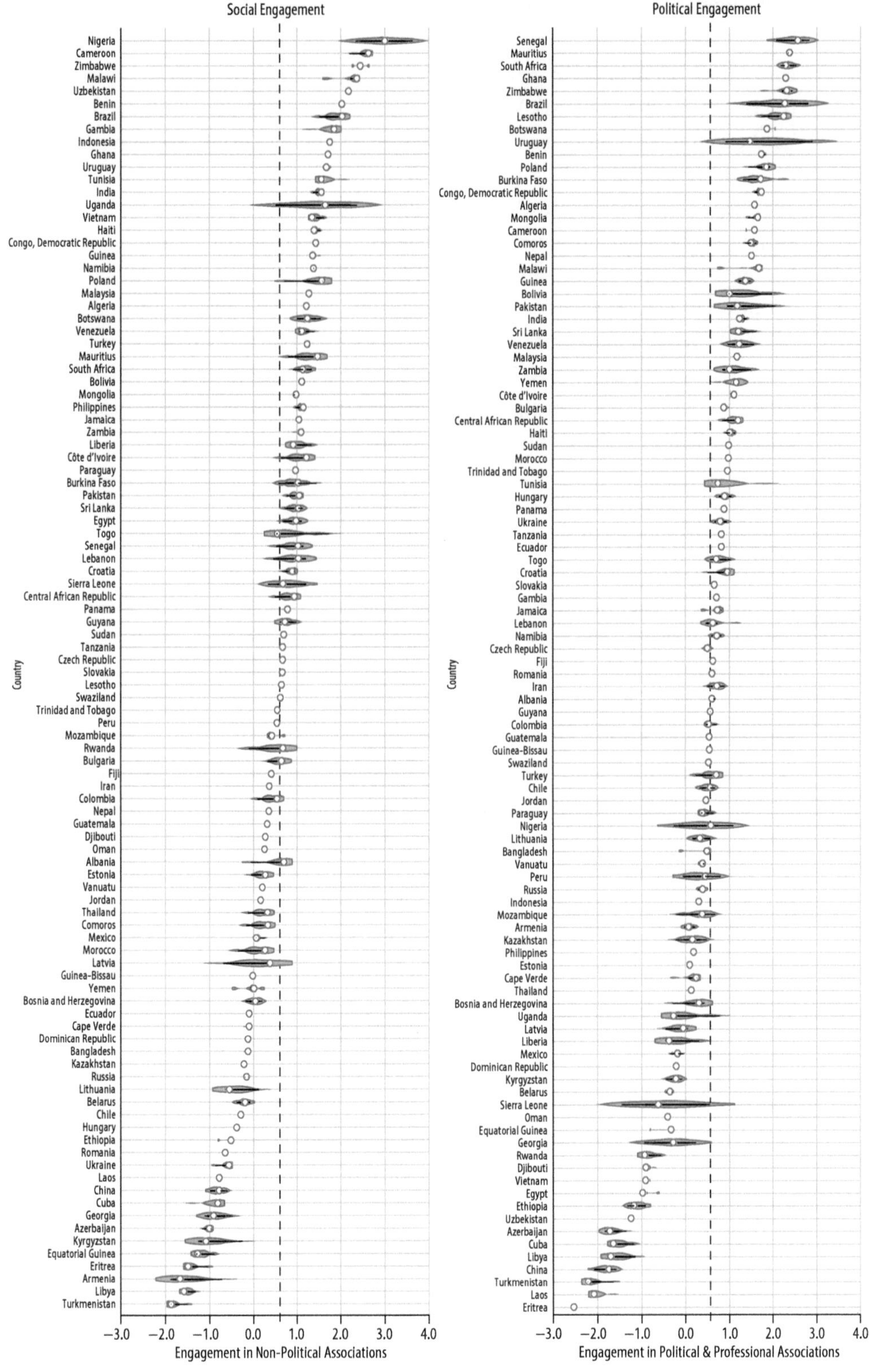

Social Engagement
Political Engagement
Country
Country
Engagement in Non-Political Associations
Engagement in Political & Professional Associations

correlation between both measures of civic engagement is moderately strong ($r = 0.6$, $N = 443$, $p < 0.001$). Within-country variation in social engagement has been highest among sub-Saharan African and Eastern European countries. In particular, citizen participation in non-political associations has changed most strongly in Uganda, Nigeria, and Latvia. In Uganda, for instance, social engagement continuously increased from 1980 onward after the end of the authoritarian rule of Idi Amin. This trend was spurred by the adoption of structural adjustment programs, which increased the number of NGOs providing essential public services. By contrast, variation is lowest in Latin America and Asia, as illustrated by countries such as Peru and Malaysia, where social engagement—at a comparatively high level—was almost constant over the entire period 1990–2015.

With regard to political participation, changes in citizen engagement have been highest in Latin America. In Uruguay, for instance, levels of engagement in political and professional associations have continuously increased, paralleled by the country's re-democratization after the end of the military regime in 1984. By contrast, within-country variation in political engagement was lowest in Asia and Eastern Europe, for instance, in Nepal and Romania.

Correlates of Social and Political Engagement

Social and political engagement are expected to improve aid effectiveness by empowering communities to voice joint concerns and engage in collective action. Communities' willingness and capacity enable citizens to participate in citizen-led accountability action, such as monitoring and evaluation activities or elite-challenging actions to hold service providers and implementing agencies accountable. The following section tests these propositions and examines the relationships between individual and country levels of civic engagement and the direct determinants of citizen demand for accountability using data from international public-opinion surveys.

To link social and political engagement with citizen action for accountability, this study draws upon the theory of planned behavior, which connects individuals' attitudes, subjective norms, and capacities with the intention to act and the action itself. According to the theory, "intention is the immediate antecedent of behavior and is itself a function of attitude toward the behavior, subjective norm, and perceived behavioral control; and these determinants follow, respectively, from beliefs about the behavior's likely consequences, about normative expectations of important others, and about the presence of factors that control behavioral performance" (Ajzen 2012, 438). Attitudes that indicate how much an individual favors citizen action for accountability are reflected by the psychological predispositions that shape a belief system supportive of liberal democratic attitudes toward political action (Klingemann 2014, 121–122). Conversely, subjective norms that indicate the perceived expectations in society to engage in cooperative behavior are reflected by the extent of reciprocity norms and levels of generalized trust. Both liberal democratic attitudes and beliefs of reciprocity interact with communities' capacity to engage in collective action and together determine citizen demand for accountability.

If social and political engagement shape citizens' willingness to exercise voice and foster communities' capacity to engage in collective action, we would observe a significant association with individuals' interest in community affairs; value orientations that put emphasis on keeping elites honest, accountable, and responsive to citizens' needs; expectations of cooperative behavior; and, ultimately, with citizens' participation in political action. The following section thus examines the proposed relationships based on data from the World Values Survey over the period 1990–2014. While international public-opinion data is available for only a smaller sample of about 60 aid recipient countries, it allows for the inspection of the proposed relationships at the individual and country level.

Regarding the relationship with citizens' willingness to engage in public matters, I first examine the reported levels of political interest. Figure 4.2 shows a statistically significant and moderately strong positive correlation between the level of citizen engagement and a country's share of respondents who evaluate politics as very important ($r = 0.35$, $N = 62$, $p < 0.005$). This relationship between political motivation and civic engagement is replicated at the individual level after accounting for country and wave fixed effects as well as for differences in sex and age (table 4.2). By implication, the presented evidence suggests civic engagement is associated with a higher interest in community affairs. Although the strength of the relationship varies, there is no difference in the nature of the relationship between different types of social and political engagement. The size of the positive association ranges from 0.2 to 0.6 standard deviations and is strongest for

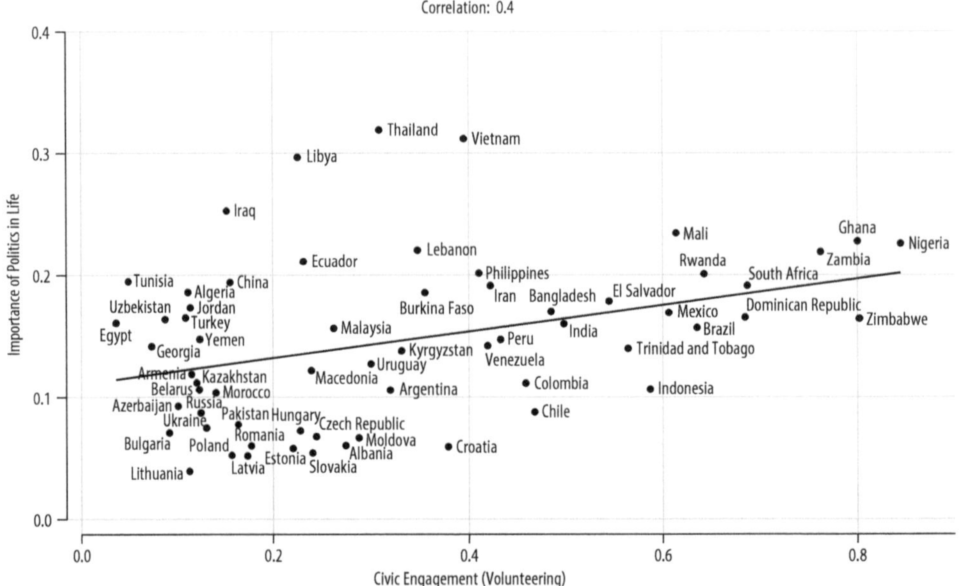

Figure 4.2. **Civic Engagement and the Importance of Politics.** *Note:* Civic engagement is measured as the percentage of respondents volunteering in at least one voluntary association. Political interest is measured as the percentage of respondents who evaluate politics as very important in their own lives.

members of political and professional organizations. The results presented in table 4.2 also show that political motivation is positively associated with engagement in elite-challenging action.

These results are also robust across varying regional and political contexts. Specifically, comparing autocracies and democracies, patronage and bureaucratic countries, as well as centralized and decentralized countries, replicates the original results.[4] In other words, there is a significant positive effect of social and political engagement on political motivation independent of countries' level of liberal democracy, state capacity, and decentralization in recipient countries.[5] Thus, regardless of a recipient country's regional or political context, social and political engagement—including elite-challenging actions—is associated with higher interest in community matters.

Political interest is one way to capture political motivation. Another is to look at the principles and ideals that motivate citizens' attitudes and behavior—in particular, individuals' willingness to keep elites honest, ac-

Table 4.2. Correlates of Social and Political Engagement

	Political Motivation	Support for Liberal Democracy	Emancipative Values	Out-Group Trust	Elite-Challenging Action
	(1)	(2)	(3)	(4)	(5)
Active civic engagement (any association)	0.26*** (0.006)	−0.01 (0.006)	0.09*** (0.005)	0.12*** (0.007)	0.34*** (0.006)
Active engagement in political and professional organizations	0.52*** (0.008)	0.10*** (0.008)	0.18*** (0.007)	0.15*** (0.010)	0.55*** (0.008)
Active engagement in leisure and welfare organizations	0.24*** (0.007)	0.10*** (0.007)	0.18*** (0.006)	0.13*** (0.008)	0.38*** (0.007)
Active engagement in religious associations	0.10*** (0.007)	−0.19*** (0.007)	−0.10*** (0.006)	0.10*** (0.009)	0.07*** (0.007)
Civic engagement (any association)	0.25*** (0.005)	0.03*** (0.006)	0.10*** (0.005)	0.09*** (0.007)	0.37*** (0.006)
Engagement in political and professional organizations	0.41*** (0.006)	0.14*** (0.006)	0.18*** (0.005)	0.13*** (0.008)	0.46*** (0.006)
Engagement in leisure and welfare organizations	0.25*** (0.006)	0.11*** (0.006)	0.19*** (0.005)	0.11*** (0.007)	0.37*** (0.006)
Engagement in religious associations	0.11*** (0.006)	−0.14*** (0.007)	−0.08*** (0.006)	0.09*** (0.008)	0.14*** (0.007)
Elite-challenging action	0.26*** (0.002)	0.126*** (0.003)	0.16*** (0.002)	0.09*** (0.004)	

(continued)

Table 4.2. Correlates of Social and Political Engagement (continued)

	Political Motivation	Support for Liberal Democracy	Emancipative Values	Out-Group Trust	Elite-Challenging Action
	(1)	(2)	(3)	(4)	(5)
Country FE	Yes	Yes	Yes	Yes	Yes
Wave FE	Yes	Yes	Yes	Yes	Yes
Sex	Yes	Yes	Yes	Yes	Yes
Age	Yes	Yes	Yes	Yes	Yes
N >=	160,376	117,101	159,039	159,039	138,474

Note: Table shows individual-level OLS estimates with country and wave fixed effects. Each outcome variable is regressed on each of the different civic-engagement measures while simultaneously accounting for age, sex, country, and wave fixed effects. Outcome variables are standardized (with a mean of 0 and a standard deviation of 1). The political motivation index summarizes how respondents evaluate the importance of politics in their own life and how much they are interested in politics (each on a 4-point scale). Support for liberal democracy is measured by adjusting the "support for democracy" index with liberal value orientations. Out-group trust is measured by averaging respondents' reported levels of trust (on a 4-point scale) in "people of another religion," "people of another nationality," and "people you meet the first time." Emancipative values are measured based on 12 items averaged into four subindices, reflecting respondents' emphasis of value orientations about freedom of choice, equality of opportunity, autonomy, and citizen voice. Active engagement indicates whether respondents reported being an active member of political and professional, leisure and welfare, or faith-based associations, respectively, or not. Elite-challenging action is measured by the Social Movement Activity index (SMA). The SMA index measures citizens' participation in elite-challenging action based on whether individuals have signed a petition, joined boycotts, or attended lawful demonstrations. *** $p < 0.01$, ** $p < 0.05$, * $p < 0.1$.

countable, and responsive to citizens' needs. If social and political engagement strengthens individuals' political motivation, we would expect to find a positive correlation between civic engagement and the extent to which citizens emphasize civic values and democratic preferences.

To measure the prevalence of civic values, I use the Emancipative Values Index (EVI), which reflects the importance an individual ascribes to freedom of choice, equality of opportunity, autonomy, and citizen voice (Welzel 2013, 57–104). To capture individuals' liberal democratic preferences, I create an index that combines respondents' support for liberal democracy with liberal value orientations (Welzel and Alexander 2017, 12–13).[6] In other words, citizens with liberal democratic preferences support liberal democracy and share liberal value orientations. While the EVI is available for the entire period under investigation, the coverage of liberal democratic preferences ranges from 1995 to 2015.

The scatterplots shown in figure 4.3 and figure 4.4 visualize the country-level relationships between political engagement in elite-challenging action and emancipative value orientations, indicating individuals' willingness to

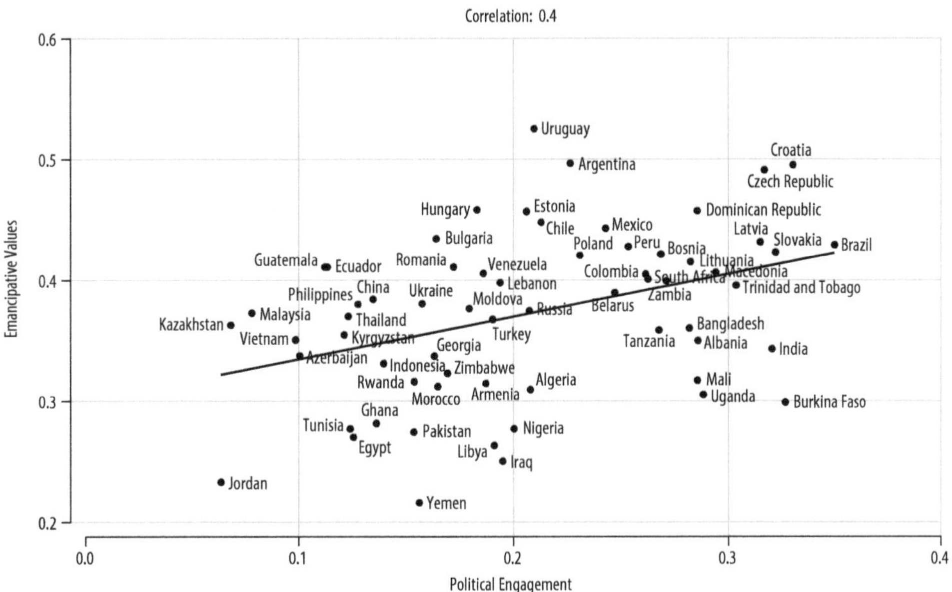

Figure 4.3. Political Engagement and Emancipative Value Orientations. *Note:* Political engagement is measured by the Social Movement Activity index.

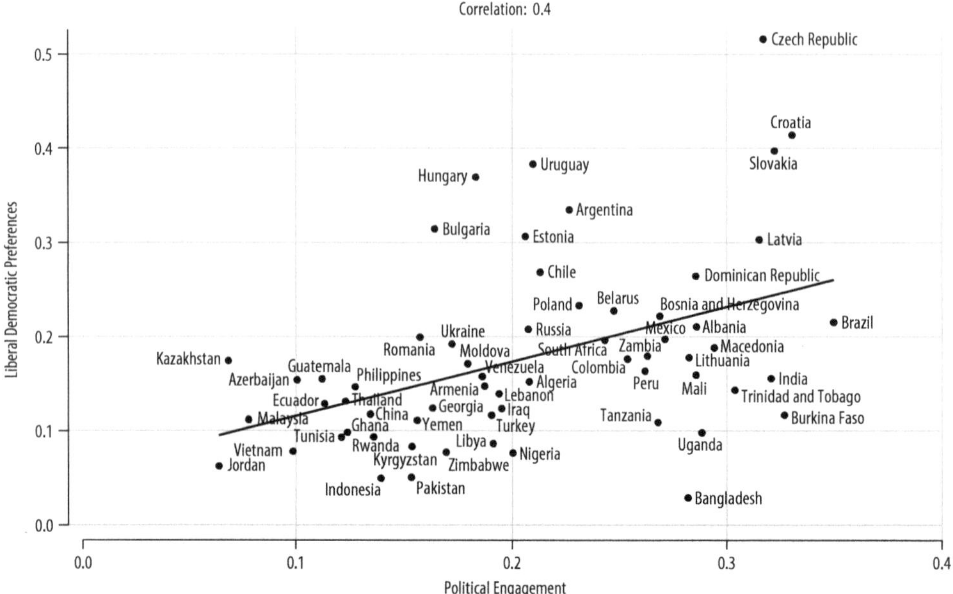

Figure 4.4. **Political Engagement and Liberal Democratic Preferences.** *Note:* Political engagement is measured by the Social Movement Activity index.

exercise voice and demand equal opportunities based on liberal democratic preferences. In particular, figure 4.3 shows a significant positive relationship between political engagement and value orientations that place emphasis on freedom of choice, equality of opportunities, and citizen voice ($r = 0.39$, $N = 63$, $p < 0.005$). Furthermore, figure 4.4 shows a significant positive association with support for liberal democracy ($r = 0.44$, $N = 61$, $p < 0.001$). Both indicate that civic values and democratic preferences are widespread in countries with higher levels of political engagement.

At the individual level, those who are politically active, including in elite-challenging actions, and those who join non-religious associations have stronger civic value orientations and show higher support for liberal democracy (table 4.2). The positive effects on civic value orientations and democratic preferences are significant, ranging from 0.1 to 0.3 standard deviations depending on the regional and political context. In contrast, compared to their non-religious counterparts, members of faith-based organizations are less supportive of emancipative values and liberal democratic orientations. Yet the observed negative correlation between religious engagement and emancipative values should be interpreted in light of the index's secular conception of emancipation. This conception emphasizes not only citizen voice and equality but also liberal freedoms, including tolerance of divorce, abortion, and homosexuality, and independence from authorities, religious or otherwise.

In conclusion, engagement in non-religious organizations and elite-challenging actions both correlate positively with democratic preferences and value orientations that emphasize freedom of choice, equality of opportunities, and citizen voice. These findings support the claim that civic engagement in aid recipient countries is linked to an increased willingness to hold political elites accountable regardless of regional and political context. For policymakers, the observed correlations underscore the potential of strengthening civic engagement in aid recipient countries, as it fosters citizens' motivation to hold authorities accountable even in challenging contexts.

Citizen action to demand accountability also depends on cooperative norms and individuals' expectations about others' participation in collective actions, such as monitoring and evaluating the provision of health and other services. Stronger generalized norms of reciprocity are expected to facilitate collective action. Thus, a positive correlation between civic engagement and out-group trust would suggest that the perceived social pressure to engage in cooperative behavior is higher in countries with an already active citizenry. This in turn can stimulate further citizen action.

To measure norms of cooperation, it is common practice to look at trust in individuals outside one's immediate social, ethnic, or religious group (Delhey, Newton, and Welzel 2011, 787). Out-group trust that bridges social cleavages and connects people of different social backgrounds is particularly likely to foster large-scale collective action. To measure out-group trust, I use an index that combines respondents' reported levels of trust in "people of another religion," "people of another nationality," and "people you meet the first time."[7] Data on out-group trust is available for 50 aid recipient countries for Wave 5 (2005–2009) and Wave 6 (2010–2014) of the WVS.

Figure 4.5 visualizes the relationship between levels of out-group trust and social engagement at the country level. The figure shows a positive, albeit weak, correlation ($r = 0.26$, $N = 50$, $p = 0.074$), suggesting that social norms of cooperation are slightly more widespread in countries with higher

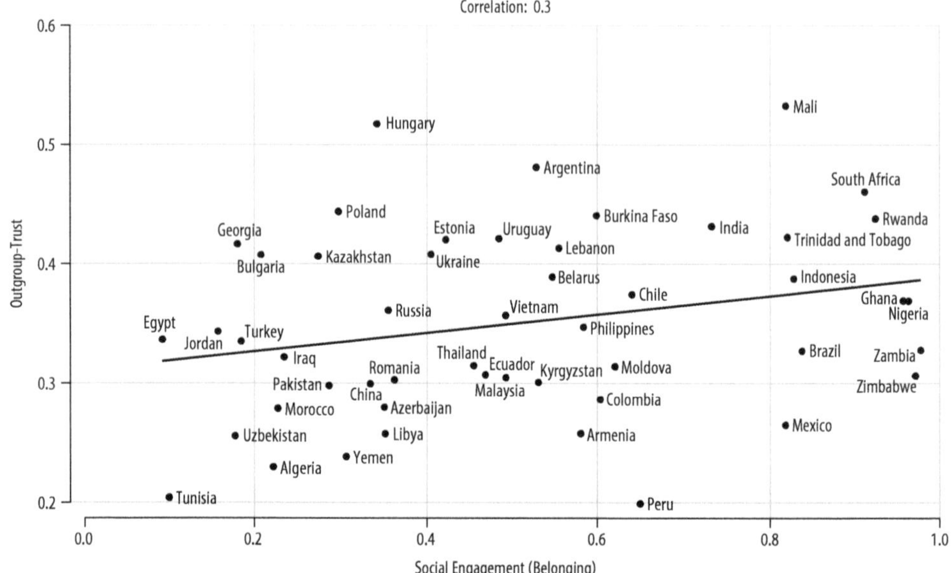

Figure 4.5. Social Engagement and Out-Group Trust. *Note:* Social engagement is measured as the percentage of respondents belonging to at least one voluntary association.

levels of social engagement. The positive correlation is also evident at the individual level, indicating that citizens who join voluntary associations have more trust in remote others (table 4.2). The same applies to individuals who engage in non-institutionalized forms of political action. The effects of social and political engagement on out-group trust are statistically and substantially significant, ranging from 0.1 to 0.3 standard deviations. Moreover, these findings are robust across diverse geographical and political contexts, indicating that social and political engagement is linked to social norms that shape individuals' expectations of cooperative behavior in recipient countries.

This interpretation is further supported by the positive correlation between social engagement and citizen participation in elite-challenging actions, as shown in figure 4.6. Countries with higher levels of social engagement tend to show greater citizen involvement in actions, such as protests and strikes. The correlation is both substantially and statistically significant ($r = 0.43$, $N = 59$, $p < 0.001$), emphasizing the direct link

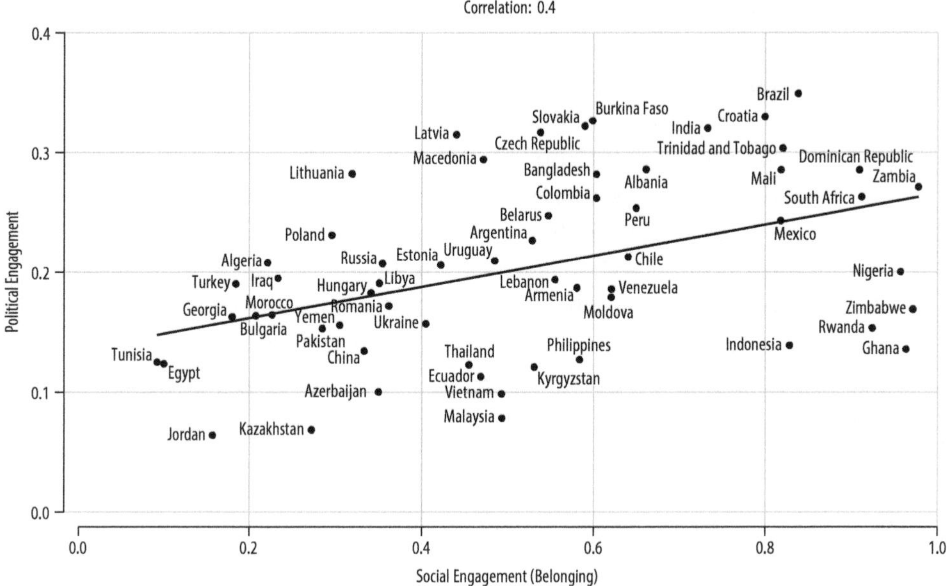

Figure 4.6. Social Engagement and Elite-Challenging Political Engagement. *Note:* Social engagement is measured as the percentage of respondents belonging to at least one voluntary association. Political engagement is measured by the Social Movement Activity index.

between social engagement and communities' capacities to exercise pressure and demand accountability. This result is also confirmed at the individual level (table 4.2). Across different regional and political contexts, social and political engagement significantly increases individuals' participation in elite-challenging action, with increases ranging from 0.2 to 0.7 standard deviations.

In summary, several factors, including political interest, civic value orientations, democratic preferences, and cooperative norms, were proposed to shape individuals' willingness and capacity to exercise voice and engage in oversight activities and elite-challenging actions. Against this backdrop, this section examined whether social and political engagement at the individual and country-level correlates with the antecedents of citizen action for accountability.

The reported evidence demonstrates that social and political engagement in aid recipient countries is positively correlated with interest in community affairs, social norms of cooperation, and participation in elite-challenging action. Furthermore, democratic preferences and value orientations that put emphasis on equal opportunities, freedom of choice, and citizen voice are significantly more widespread among citizens engaged in non-religious voluntary associations. Conversely, engagement in faith-based organizations is not associated with such liberal social values or democratic orientations but is still linked to higher interest in political matters, cooperative norms, and engagement in elite-challenging actions. Similarly, citizens who engage in accountability actions share a strong interest in politics, democratic preferences, civic value orientations, and norms of cooperation, equipping them with the motivation and capacity to hold political authorities accountable.

It is noteworthy that the relationships between citizen engagement and individuals' motivation and capacity to demand accountability are similar for active and passive members of voluntary associations. The intensity of voluntary engagement thus only plays a minor role. Furthermore, the identified linkages between civic engagement and citizen demand for accountability are consistent across different geographical regions and political contexts. Overall, social and political engagement in aid recipient countries increases communities' willingness to voice concerns of public interest and their capacity to engage in citizen-led actions to demand accountability.

The Coevolution of Health Aid, Civic Engagement, and Infant Mortality

Based on the observed effects of civic engagement on citizen demand for accountability and the proposition that performance oversight makes aid work better, we expect the correlation between health aid and population health to vary across different levels of civic engagement. Simply put, if aid is effective, more health funding will be followed by declines in infant mortality in later periods. And if this relationship depends on the presence of a vibrant voluntary sector, this negative association will be more evident in countries with high citizen engagement. Conversely, in societies with weaker civil-society participation, the link will be less pronounced. Figure 4.7 illustrates this relationship by comparing annual changes in health aid per capita and infant mortality for a set of recipient countries with varying levels of social engagement.

Figure 4.7 shows the moving average of lagged levels of health aid per capita (log scale) and infant mortality (log scale) for a set of countries with active or largely inactive voluntary sectors, defined by social engagement levels one standard deviation above vs. below the mean or higher.[8] Among the countries with high citizen engagement, there is a clear negative relationship between lagged health aid and subsequent infant mortality. For instance, in Mali and Vietnam, the correlation between aid and the mortality rate is −0.6 and −0.9, respectively, indicating that previous increases in health aid commitments tend to be followed by declines in infant mortality. Consistent with the proposed theory, this shows that a vibrant voluntary sector is associated with a striking negative relationship between lagged health aid and infant mortality.

In contrast, countries with below-average levels of social engagement display no clear relationship between health aid and public health. The correlation within countries is close to zero or even positive, as in Panama and Iran, implying that in less engaged societies, health aid does not necessarily equate to improved population health.

It is important to note the diverse political contexts of the countries shown in figure 4.7. While the countries have been selected primarily based on their varying levels of civic engagement, their differences in population health, aid, and political-context factors make the sample selection less prone to unmeasured confounding.[9] For instance, societies with a vibrant voluntary sector range from countries with high mortality rates, such as Mali and Malawi, to those with lower rates, like Vietnam and Indonesia. The sample is also diverse concerning the extent of aid dependency and institutional quality. More-aid-dependent countries include centralized patronage autocracies like Zimbabwe and decentralized democracies like Tanzania. By contrast, among less-aid-dependent countries, the political context varies from centralized bureaucratic autocracies like Vietnam to decentralized patronage democracies like Ghana.

In summary, the observed trends of health aid and population health across these diverse countries support the proposed moderating impact of citizen engagement on aid effectiveness. These insights should be viewed as suggestive evidence that requires further testing, however, and not as representative of the entire sample of recipient countries.

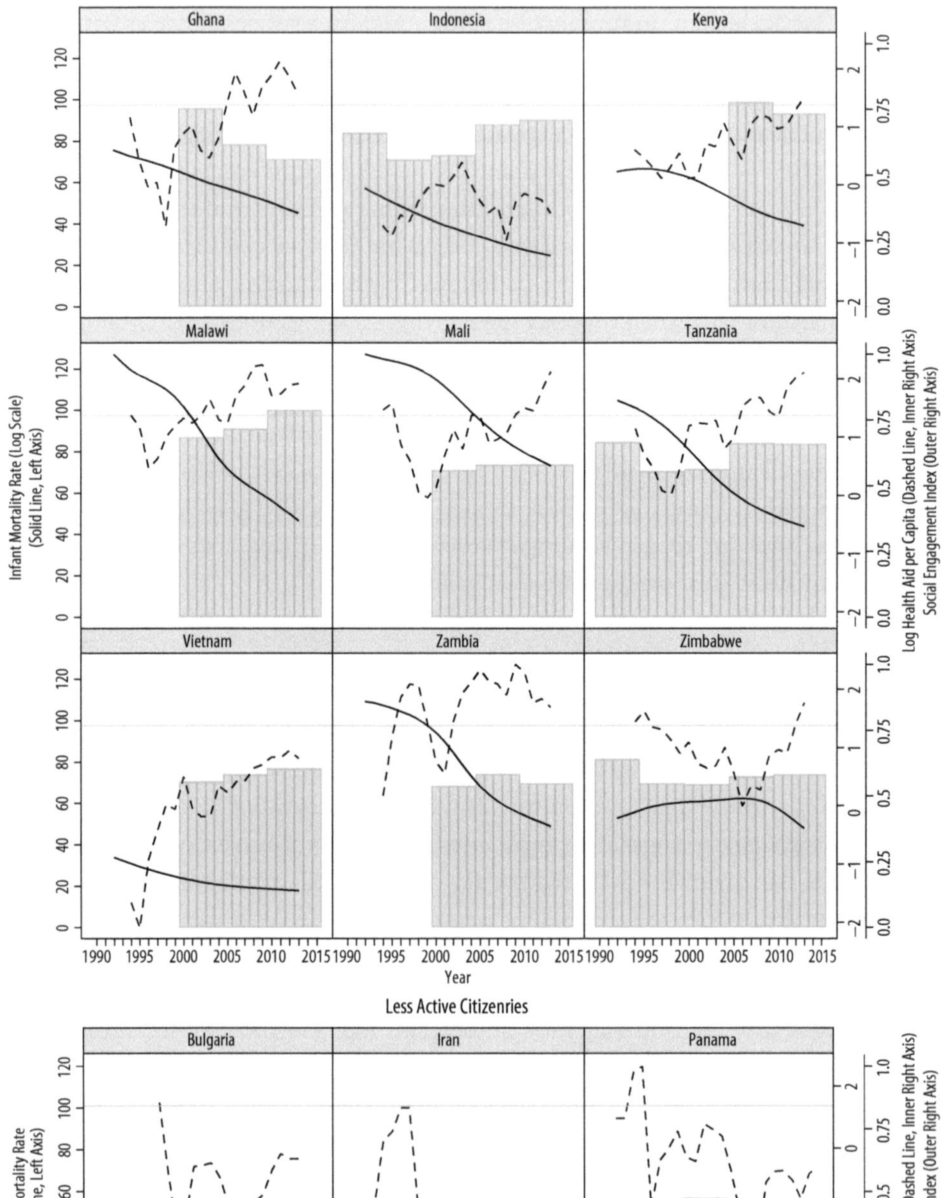

Highly Active Citizenries
Ghana
Indonesia
Kenya
Malawi
Mali
Tanzania
Vietnam
Zambia
Zimbabwe
Infant Mortality Rate (Log Scale)
(Solid Line, Left Axis)
Log Health Aid per Capita (Dashed Line, Inner Right Axis)
Social Engagement Index (Outer Right Axis)
Year
Less Active Citizenries
Bulgaria
Iran
Panama
Infant Mortality Rate
(Solid Line, Left Axis)
Log Health Aid per Capita (Dashed Line, Inner Right Axis)
Social Engagement Index (Outer Right Axis)
Year

Case-Study Evidence

The following section provides case-study evidence to illustrate the importance of ordinary citizens' engagement in community organizations for mobilizing citizen action and demanding accountability from public authorities in the health sector. The insights of these studies deepen not only our understanding of health interventions that seek to strengthen citizen demands for accountability but also shed light on how the structure of community ties conditions the success of donor-funded health interventions in general.

The first multiple case study by Hernández et al. (2020) explores the role of networks in citizen-led health accountability initiatives at the municipal level in Guatemala. The health system in Guatemala is characterized by high maternal mortality rates and chronic malnutrition among children under five, especially among Indigenous communities. The quality of public health can be partly attributed to the state's lack of organizational and decision-making capacities essential to coordinate health services, mobilize resources, and implement health processes. As a result, the country has received, on average, about $34 million in health aid annually between 1990 and 2013. The decentralized nature of the health system gives health officials at the regional level some administrative and decision-making authority over the planning, coordination, and evaluation of health programs. Public officials at the municipal level are responsible for managing and distributing funds for health-care services and overseeing service delivery.

Under these conditions, the Center for the Study of Equity and Governance in Health Systems (CEGSS), a local civil-society organization, was funded by international donors to support accountability initiatives that redress the causes of health inequalities and promote better health-system

---

Figure 4.7. *(opposite)* **Active vs. Inactive Citizenries and the Coevolution of Health Aid and Infant Mortality.** *Note:* The figure shows the moving average of lagged health aid per capita (log scale) and infant mortality (log scale) over time for selected countries with high vs. low levels of social engagement (one standard deviation above or below the mean). Averages are calculated over five-year periods, with decreasing weights for more recent health aid commitments and equal weights for mortality levels. The dotted horizontal line indicates the average level of health aid per capita across all aid recipient countries. Bar graphs show average levels of the Social Engagement Index.

governance in rural communities of Guatemala.[10] To mobilize citizen action for accountability, the implementing organization provided ongoing training and support to volunteering community members (civic activists) in several municipalities. The aim was to enable civic activists to organize visits to health-care facilities to monitor service delivery, gather feedback from health-service users about their experiences, and engage with authorities at various levels to advocate for potential solutions.[11] In each municipality, the activists collaborated—as a citizen-led initiative—with community authorities (village leaders) and various members of community associations, including women's community-based organizations, agricultural cooperatives, rural community organizations, urban civil-society associations, and traditional birth-attendant organizations. Three municipalities were selected to study the role of community ties as determinants of effective civic activism in further detail using network mapping and interpretive analysis (Hernández et al. 2020).

The study documents that the civic activists, in cooperation with their network of community organizations, were able to effectively monitor and document a wide range of problems related to service delivery, including poor health infrastructure, lack of medicines, and cases of abuse and mistreatment in the district hospital. Against this backdrop, the activists engaged with public authorities at various levels, demanding improvements in medicine supply and health infrastructure, and resolution to grievances related to maltreatment and discrimination. Specifically, activists regularly participated in the municipal council, presented petitions initiated with the support of their collaborators and community networks, and contacted authorities at various levels, including mayors, health district managers, regional health directors, ombudspersons, public prosecutors, and provincial and national officials. In one municipality, the activists maintained regular contact with the vice minister of health about the availability of medicines in the health posts. In another municipality, the activists filed a collective grievance at a regional anti-discrimination office to address the abuse and maltreatment of traditional birth attendants and their patients in the hospital.

The initiative led to modest improvements in health-service delivery and government responsiveness. In two cases, the initiatives gained influence and mobilized additional municipal resources to improve the health infrastructure and medicine supply. Furthermore, the coordination between municipal and district health authorities was improved. Yet, in one case, the initiative failed to obtain a response from the local authorities despite presenting substantial evidence of rights violations and discrimination in service delivery and the support of local community organizations. Overall, the authors point to the importance of relational ties in empowering citizens to improve health-sector accountability and how network resources can facilitate shifting the power balance between the state and citizens in contexts of weak state capacity.

In one of the three municipalities, the mix of weak and strong relational ties with community members who were able and willing to communicate with the local population and lend their influence to petitions enabled the initiative's work to gain recognition and credibility. In the second case, the initiative benefited from a network of mostly weak ties connecting citizen leaders that gave voice mainly to rural service users' problems with civic activists who regularly exercised pressure and demanded accountability from authorities at different levels. The third case illustrates how collaborative ties between urban-based activists and community organizations enabled the initiative to reach service users, expose and document abusive and discriminatory treatment, and activate vertical accountability mechanisms by collaborating with a national representative of an anti-discrimination office.

In sum, the activists successfully mobilized collective accountability action and connected political authorities with constituencies. The study highlights the crucial role of community associations in connecting activists (who received training and support funded by development assistance) with different population segments, raising awareness, and bringing together users of rural services who experience health-system failures. The study's authors further conclude that the communities' relational ties were "fundamental to their ability to mobilize collective action to give voice and demand attention to rural health system failures. This grassroots support helped the citizen-led initiatives gain recognition and legitimacy as representatives of the people" (Hernández et al. 2020, 13).

Another multiple case study by Mafuta et al. (2016) examines the role of context factors in facilitating citizen demand for accountability in the Moanda and Bolenge health zones in the Democratic Republic of the Congo. The study highlights the importance of cultural and political context conditions as necessary to improving maternal health and ensuring the effectiveness of donor-funded health interventions.

The health system in the fragile and conflict-affected Democratic Republic of the Congo (DRC) is characterized by one of the highest maternal mortality ratios worldwide. The high mortality among mothers stems from limited access to reproductive health services, malnutrition, infectious diseases, and ongoing armed conflicts. The public-health situation is also related to the state's incapacity to deliver essential services, implement health policies, and manage conflicts. To support the poor-quality health system, between 1990 and 2013, the DRC received annual health aid from international donors averaging about $212 million.

Against this backdrop, the authors of this study examined the role of cultural and political context factors in Moanda and Bolenge, where partner organizations implemented health interventions that targeted maternal health through different project-based activities, including strengthening citizen-led accountability action (Mafuta et al. 2015, 3). The Moanda health zone, situated in the western region of the DRC in the affluent province of Kongo Central, serves approximately 137,000 residents through its 9 health centers. The Bolenge health zone, located in the northwestern Équateur province—one of the poorest in the DRC—provides services to about 80,000 residents with its 15 health centers.[12] To examine how the cultural and political context enables or constrains individuals to voice their concerns regarding health services and to be mobilized into collective accountability actions, the authors conducted interviews with community actors in both health zones, including public officials, health-service providers, and community representatives.

The interviews revealed that despite the presence of multiple community organizations, the cultural context of both health zones was unfavorable to and not supportive of implementing health interventions that require citizen action for accountability. In particular, the authors find that community groups were focused mainly on their core activities and rarely engaged in collective actions related to the provision of public goods and health services. The study finds that a lack of knowledge and skills to mobilize accountability action among members of community organizations; the absence of coalitions and alliances between groups, external NGOs, and governmental bodies; and the perceived lack of responsiveness from health providers and public authorities limited users' capacity and willingness to make demands (Mafuta et al. 2015, 6). Furthermore, the dominance of patriarchal values (favoring early marriage) restricted women's access to education and work opportunities, and hindered women's autonomy and participation in making demands to improve health-service delivery. Additional sociocultural factors included the presence of tensions between groups of different ethnic origins, the absence of radio broadcasting or television that provided health-related information to a large number of community members, and the low interest in the community's health affairs, including the performance of health-service providers.

Concerning the political context, the study's authors find that despite a constitutional mandate for the devolution of power to local authorities, decision-making related to health-service delivery took place at the central level. The absence of locally elected decision-makers thus limited service users' opportunities to have a say in the planning and implementation of service delivery and lowered public officials' motivation to respond to the needs of local constituents. The local political context in both health zones also limited community groups' opportunities to demand accountability as they required authorization from political authorities in order to hold public meetings and implement activities. Community groups advocating for accountability and better service provision were even subject to repressive measures. Additionally, community groups were subject to vote buying and electoral clientelism to ensure political support during elections. Furthermore, the study shows that health committee members who monitored the quality of service delivery and the performance of health centers were not freely elected and thus lacked legitimacy.

To conclude, the authors' assessment of the cultural and political contexts in both health zones of the Democratic Republic of the Congo suggests they were not conducive to health interventions that rely on citizen demands for accountability (Mafuta et al. 2016, 10). The study shows the importance of the cultural context and how the absence of inter-group relationships and networks for collective action that can bridge social and ethnic divides, as well as civic values that put emphasis on equality and voice, can undermine citizens' capacity and motivation to demand accountability from public authorities and service providers. The study also highlights the role of the political context and demonstrates that the absence of decentralized decision-making processes and the lack of formal institutions that guarantee the freedom of expression and association and foster an independent media constrain health interventions that depend on citizen action for accountability.

To summarize, this chapter has outlined differences in levels of social and political engagement across diverse regional and political contexts. Sub-Saharan Africa and Latin America, the regions that have received the largest amounts of health aid, have the highest levels of civic engagement. Eastern Europe and the MENA region maintain the lowest levels of citizen engagement. Exploiting this variation in associational involvement, the chapter provides evidence that citizen engagement in voluntary organizations is associated with higher interest in community affairs, stronger norms of cooperation, and greater participation in citizen-led accountability actions. Furthermore, excluding faith-based organizations, associational involvement is also linked to liberal democratic preferences and value orientations that put emphasis on freedom of choice, equal opportunities, and citizen voice. Together, these results suggest that social and political engagement in aid recipient countries strengthens the willingness and the capacity to voice shared concerns and exercise pressure on public authorities, enabling citizen action for accountability.

Resting on a broader data basis, the findings challenge previous claims that associational involvement suppresses regime-threatening forms of protest activity and stabilizes authoritarian leaders. Instead, civic engagement appears to strengthen citizen demand for accountability across varying political contexts, even in the least democratic settings.

Comparing a set of selected countries with more or less active citizenries, the last part of the chapter explores the coevolution of health aid and population health and employs multiple case studies that shed light on the mechanisms linking associational networks with aid and public-health outcomes. The evidence illustrates civic engagement's pivotal role in making aid work and highlights the importance of community associations to mobilize collective action and demand accountability in health-care delivery. The next section will test the relationship from a dynamic and multilevel perspective to account for endogeneity issues.

NOTES

1. In sub-Saharan Africa, members actively involved in religious organizations consist of 39.7 percent Protestants, 22 percent Roman Catholics, 14.6 percent Muslims, and 23 percent from other religious denominations. Across all regions, active religious membership comprises Roman Catholics at 34 percent, Protestants at 22 percent, Muslims 13 percent, Hindus 4 percent, and 26 percent from other religious denominations.

2. For a comprehensive discussion of relevant factors contributing to the emergence and unfolding of the Arab Spring, see Ardic (2012).

3. By contrast, using data on international NGO density and social-movement activity, Foa and Ekiert (2017) argue that civil societies in Central and Eastern European countries are not as weak as commonly assumed since many post-communist countries maintain an active civil-society sector that is strongly connected to transnational civic networks and able to shape domestic policies.

4. Countries are classified as patronage, semi-patronage, and bureaucratic countries based on the ordinal version of V-Dem's public-sector corruption index. The three-point scale measures the extent to which public-sector employees misappropriate public resources for private use.

Regimes are classified based on the Democracy vs. Dictatorship index introduced by Cheibub, Gandhi, and Vreeland (2010). According to this index, a regime is considered a democracy if the executive and the legislature are directly or indirectly elected by popular vote, multiple parties are allowed and exist (outside the regime), there are multiple parties within the legislature, and there has been no consolidation of incumbent advantage (e.g., unconstitutional closing of the lower house or extension of incumbent's term by postponing subsequent elections).

Countries are classified as administratively and politically decentralized according to whether subnational governments have extensive taxing, spending, or regulatory authority and whether state or provincial governments (or both) are locally elected. The estimates of the subgroup analyses are not shown but are available upon request from the author.

5. The only exception to this general pattern is the insignificant correlation between social engagement in faith-based organizations in Eastern Europe and societies classified as bureaucratic countries.

6. The index of "liberal democratic preferences" is calculated by multiplying the "support for liberal democracy" and the "liberal values" subindex. In particular, the "support for democracy" index averages respondents' preferences for "Having a democratic political system," disagreement with "Having the army rule," and disagreement with "Having a strong leader who does not have to bother with parliaments and elections" (each on a 4-point scale). The variables are recoded into a range from 0 to 1, with decimal fractions of 1 indicating intermediate positions. Each respondent's position over the three items is then averaged to build the "support for democracy" index ranging from 0 (strongly rejecting democracy and strongly supporting the army rule/strong leaders) to 1 (the exact opposite position).

The resulting index is multiplied by liberal sexuality values, including respondents' tolerance of homosexuality, abortion, and divorce, to capture the liberal notions of democratic support. These 10-point scales are recoded into a range from 0 (never justifiable) to 1 (always justifiable), with decimal fractions of 1 indicating intermediate positions. Each respondent's position is averaged over the three items to construct a liberal values subindex. Country-level scores are population averages on this 0-to-1 scale.

7. Each 4-point scale ranges from "Do not trust at all" to "Trust completely," and is normalized with a minimum of 0 and a maximum of 1. The average across the normalized three items is the out-group trust index. The measurement of generalized trust has

been shown to be equivalent and comparable across different cultural contexts (Freitag and Bauer 2013).

8. Average levels of health aid are calculated over five-year periods with decreasing weights for more recent commitments to account for the fact that aid is likely to affect population health with a certain time lag.

9. Despite these differences, the selected countries all fall within the range of one standard deviation around the global mean of health aid, liberal democracy, and bureaucratic governance, respectively (table A3.2).

10. Funding was provided by various international donors, including the UK Department for International Development (Hernández et al. 2020, 13; Schaaf et al. 2018, 183).

11. The implementing organization has also been active in other activities, including strengthening grassroots associations, raising public awareness about health-related entitlements, collecting information on citizen preferences and experiences with service providers, holding community assemblies, and engaging with authorities at multiple levels of the health system to advocate for action (Schaaf et al. 2018).

12. The Democratic Republic of the Congo is divided into 516 health zones. A health zone encompasses 10–20 health areas, with a health center offering services to multiple villages. Health centers are monitored by health committees, which discuss health issues at regular meetings based on reports from community health workers (Mafuta et al. 2015).

5

The Moderating Role of Civic Engagement

Does civic engagement enhance health aid effectiveness? The previous chapter established that social and political engagement are associated with an array of factors that determine communities' motivation and capacity to demand accountability, including higher interest in community affairs, stronger norms of cooperation, and value orientations that emphasize citizen voice and equal opportunities. It further demonstrated that engagement in voluntary associations is linked to greater participation in citizen-led accountability actions. These findings support the claim that active citizens are more willing and better able to hold public officials and service providers accountable. Building on these insights, the following chapter tests whether the benefits of civic engagement translate into higher aid effectiveness in countries where citizens are actively engaged in communal activities and citizen-led accountability actions.

To examine the influence of social and political engagement across countries, this study applies different estimation techniques, including GMM estimation and Heckman's two-stage selection model. These techniques account for the simultaneity of the allocation of aid to recipient countries and its potential effects on public health, and they consider non-aid-recipient countries to avoid selectivity bias. The identified effects of civic engagement are then compared with the impact of formal oversight mechanisms that have been at the center of political economists' interest, including the role of bureaucratic governance and democratic institutions. This allows us to directly compare the effects of formal political institutions vs. informal institutions shaped by community relations. The last part of this chapter tests the expected relationships among individuals from different aid recipient countries, employing multilevel analyses. The multilevel approach exploits variation within recipient countries and eliminates differences linked to features of the political and socioeconomic context. The analyses reported in this chapter provide systematic evidence supporting the claim that bottom-up rather than top-down mechanisms of accountability enhance the effects of health aid on individual and public-health outcomes.

Population Health and Aid Effectiveness: Cross-National Evidence
Social Engagement

In societies with high levels of social engagement, citizens often participate in non-political associations, engage in voluntary activities, and spend time on unpaid community work. The previous chapter highlighted that, in these vibrant societies, civic values are widespread, citizens are more interested in public matters, and they are also more likely to cooperate and engage in citizen-led actions for accountability. Thus, associational involvement in diverse social networks likely bolsters citizens' motivation to participate in community-related development interventions and provides the connective resources for mobilizing citizen action for accountability. The following section delves into whether this increased citizen motivation and capacity to demand accountability make health interventions in recipient countries more effective. Using dynamic panel data analyses, this section examines the role of social engagement in making aid improve health outcomes while controlling for a wide range of socioeconomic and sociopolitical public-health determinants. The results are presented in the table below.

Table 5.1 reports the estimated effects of social engagement and development assistance for health (DAH) on infant mortality across different indicators of non-political engagement. Across all model specifications, the negative sign of the DAH coefficient indicates a mortality-reducing effect of health aid in countries with average social engagement levels. This negative effect of health aid is robust to various sets of controls and significant except for Models 5–6 based on the smaller World Values Survey (WVS) sample. Importantly, the validity of the instruments used in all SYS-GMM models is confirmed by Hansen's-J test and implies the endogeneity of aid is properly addressed. The test for autocorrelation also indicates the absence of second-order serial correlation, which means the estimated coefficients are not rendered inconsistent.

Table 5.1. Social Engagement, Health Aid, and Population Health

	Dependent Variable: Infant Mortality Rate (Log Scale)							
	CSO Participatory Environment		Non-Political Engagement		Membership in Leisure and Welfare Associations		Social Engagement Index	
	(1)	(2)	(3)	(4)	(5)	(6)	(7)	(8)
DAH (log scale)	−0.029***	−0.025***	−0.018*	−0.018**	−0.036	−0.024	−0.027***	−0.025***
	(0.008)	(0.007)	(0.010)	(0.009)	(0.028)	(0.017)	(0.010)	(0.009)
Social engagement	−0.003	0.007	0.034	0.027	0.320	0.338*	0.353*	0.393***
	(0.018)	(0.016)	(0.024)	(0.021)	(0.241)	(0.191)	(0.202)	(0.146)
DAH (log scale) * Social engagement	−0.014***	−0.014***	−0.018*	−0.016*	−0.224**	−0.206*	−0.241**	−0.240**
	(0.004)	(0.005)	(0.010)	(0.009)	(0.110)	(0.121)	(0.120)	(0.100)
Public-sector corruption control	−0.007	0.020	−0.293**	−0.260**	−0.059	0.018	−0.109	−0.089
	(0.119)	(0.082)	(0.140)	(0.126)	(0.229)	(0.143)	(0.117)	(0.098)
Government health expenditures		−0.009**		−0.004		−0.006*		0.001
		(0.005)		(0.006)		(0.004)		(0.004)
IMR (lagged)	1.093***	1.037***	1.030***	1.018***	0.803***	0.789***	1.096***	1.081***
	(0.047)	(0.052)	(0.048)	(0.048)	(0.103)	(0.109)	(0.046)	(0.045)
Constant	0.000	0.030	0.000	−0.041	0.000	0.463	−0.554*	−0.593*
	(0.000)	(0.480)	(0.000)	(0.506)	(0.000)	(0.884)	(0.313)	(0.317)
Conflict	Yes	Yes	Yes	Yes	Yes	Yes	Yes	Yes
GDP per capita (log scale)	Yes	Yes	Yes	Yes	Yes	Yes	Yes	Yes
Population (log scale)	Yes	Yes	Yes	Yes	Yes	Yes	Yes	Yes
Fertility rate (log scale)	Yes	Yes	Yes	Yes	Yes	Yes	Yes	Yes

(continued)

Table 5.1. Social Engagement, Health Aid, and Population Health (continued)

	Dependent Variable: Infant Mortality Rate (Log Scale)							
	CSO Participatory Environment		Non-Political Engagement		Membership in Leisure and Welfare Associations		Social Engagement Index	
	(1)	(2)	(3)	(4)	(5)	(6)	(7)	(8)
Physicians (log scale)	Yes	Yes	Yes	Yes	Yes	Yes	Yes	Yes
Female education (log scale)	Yes	Yes			Yes	Yes		
Period FE	Yes	Yes	Yes	Yes	Yes	Yes	Yes	Yes
Observations	342	339	335	332	88	88	236	233
Countries	101	100	101	100	51	51	77	76
Instruments	86	91	77	82	40	42	80	85
Hansen-test	0.241	0.248	0.138	0.166	0.329	0.624	0.283	0.582
AR2	0.141	0.235	0.852	0.767			0.516	0.580

Note: Table shows two-step GMM estimation with Windmeijer bias-corrected robust standard errors. Health aid (DAH) is lagged by one period. Social engagement is measured by the CSO Participatory Environment index (Models 1–2), Non-Political Engagement index (Models 3–4), membership in leisure and welfare associations index (Models 5–6), and the Social Engagement Index (Models 7–8). DAH and social engagement are mean-centered.
*** p<0.01, ** p<0.05, * p<0.1.

Notably, across all model specifications, the interaction coefficient is negative and significant, implying the effect of increased health aid on infant mortality differs across observed levels of social engagement. Specifically, as the main and interaction effects have the same (negative) sign (Model 1), each social engagement and health aid per capita improves population health, yet together they produce a stronger effect than either would alone. This synergistic relationship implies that health aid per capita is more effective in reducing infant mortality in countries with higher levels of social engagement.

The identified enhancing effect is replicated using different measures of social engagement. These include expert ratings and international public-opinion data, as detailed in table 5.1. Models 1–4 measure social engagement using V-Dem's Participatory Environment and Non-Political Engagement index. The interaction with health aid is highly negative and significant for both measures. Using survey data on individuals' membership in leisure and welfare associations from the WVS further supports the finding that social engagement enhances the negative effect of health aid on infant mortality (Models 5–6). This result is also replicated using the Social Engagement Index, an aggregate measure of citizen participation in voluntary activities and community work (Models 7–8).

To better understand the identified interaction relationships, figure 5.1 visualizes the effects of lagged health aid on infant mortality across different levels and measures of social engagement, as detailed in table 5.1. Each plot shows that the marginal effect of health aid is insignificant in countries with low levels of social engagement. Where voluntary engagement flourishes, however, health aid significantly reduces infant mortality. These findings hold regardless of whether social engagement is measured as (A) participatory environment, (B) non-political engagement, (C) participation in leisure and welfare associations, or (D) participation in voluntary activities and community work.

Specifically, using the estimates of Models 1–2, we can infer that the effect of health aid is insignificant in places with citizen involvement below the bottom quantile. Yet, at higher levels of social engagement, the effect of increased health aid on infant mortality is significantly negative. For instance, doubling health aid per capita in a society with moderate associational involvement, like Russia in the late 1990s, would reduce infant mortality by about 3 percent. In this context, freedoms of assembly were

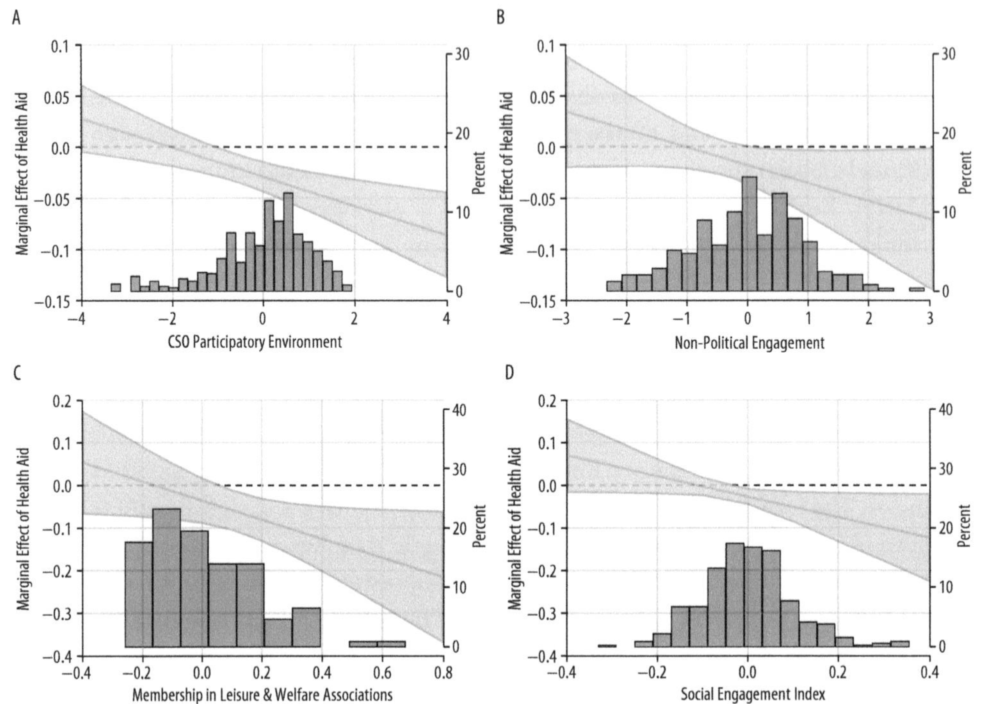

Figure 5.1. Social Engagement and the Marginal Effect of Health Aid. *Note:* Figure shows the average marginal effects of lagged health aid on infant mortality (with 95 percent confidence interval) based on two-step system GMM estimations for different measures of social engagement. Each plot visualizes the estimated effects of lagged health aid across observed levels of (A) the CSO Participatory Environment index, (B) the Non-Political Engagement index, (C) membership in leisure and welfare associations, as well as (D) citizens' participation in voluntary activities and community work. Estimates are based on Models 1, 3, 5, and 7 reported in table 5.1.

generally respected, and many diverse civil-society organizations existed, although only with moderate popular participation (Karatnycky 1999, 383–387). By contrast, in a country with an active citizenry, like Ecuador in the 1990s, with levels of social engagement one standard deviation above the mean, doubling health aid would reduce infant mortality by nearly 5 percent.[1]

According to the estimates based on the WVS sample (figure 5.1C), the enhancing effect of citizen participation in leisure and welfare associations is even larger. At levels of active citizen participation one standard deviation above the mean, doubling health aid per capita would reduce infant mortality by about 7.9 percent. This level of social engagement is similar to the one observed in Zimbabwe in the early 2010s, where nearly half the population reported belonging to at least one leisure and welfare association, and about one-quarter reported being an active member.

Overall, comparing the effect of doubling health aid in countries with moderately vs. highly active citizenries suggests that a one-standard-deviation increase in social engagement would almost double the decline in infant mortality resulting from increased health aid. These results imply that social engagement has enormous potential to make health aid work better, which lends support to Hypothesis 1a, discussed in chapter 2, which states that social engagement enhances aid effectiveness.

ROBUSTNESS CHECK

The synergistic interaction effect of social engagement is robust regardless of the chosen measure of non-political engagement and holds even after controlling for alternative explanatory factors, including different socio-economic and sociopolitical conditions.[2]

Specifically, the models consider differences in economic development, population size, conflict involvement, and public-sector corruption. These controls take into account that poorer countries receive more foreign aid and have higher mortality levels. They also factor in that population size and public-sector corruption may determine the amount of foreign aid allocated based on the number of people in need or donors' strategic behavior. Furthermore, they address the effects of violent conflicts and misappropriation of health resources by public officials.

In addition, the models consider the role of governments' domestic health expenditures and the size of the health workforce. These controls allow disentangling the impact of the initial quality of a country's health infrastructure and the effects of domestic health spending, particularly if foreign aid is primarily delivered through NGOs and multilateral organizations to bypass recipient governments with weak state institutions.

Furthermore, the results hold after accounting for the state of reproductive health care (with fertility as a proxy) and women's education. Both factors are likely to decrease infant mortality by enabling parents to devote more resources to each child and giving women better access to health services, greater empowerment, and economic independence.

I also performed a series of robustness tests to account for the role of international NGOs. World polity theory posits that countries deeply integrated in the global net of international NGOs (INGOs) are more likely to adopt global models and organizational standards, including those related to funding for public services (Paxton, Hughes, and Reith 2015, 287). Likewise, feminist-movement scholars emphasize that the global spread of women's international NGOs, or WINGOs, has increased the diffusion of norms and standards of gender equality, promoting social change in favor of women (Hughes et al. 2018, 1–2). The inherent link to reproductive health care makes WINGOs also a relevant control variable for the study of public-health outcomes. To evaluate the potential influence of INGO network integration on public-health outcomes, I use the INGO Network Country Score provided by Paxton, Hughes, and Reith (2015) as an additional control variable. This measure captures a country's centrality within the global network of international NGOs and reflects the level of connectedness to the world polity. To account for the potential role of women's international organizing on public-health outcomes, I use data from Melanie Hughes and colleagues (2018) on countries' memberships in WINGOs.[3]

Controlling for these diverse factors ensures that the estimated effects of citizen engagement and aid on public health are not confounded. Using time lags further ensures that foreign aid received in the current period is linked to health outcomes in the future and thus accounts for the fact that aid needs time to unfold its impact on public health.

Political Engagement

In politically active societies, citizens frequently engage in political associations and elite-challenging actions, aiming to exert political influence. As outlined in the previous chapter, involvement in political associations and participation in elite-challenging actions in aid recipient countries is underpinned by increased interest in community affairs, norms of cooperation, and values emphasizing citizen voice and equality in opportunities. Political engagement should thus not only shape citizens' motivation to participate in development projects affecting their communities but also enable communities to engage in oversight activities and hold providers and officials accountable to citizen preferences. The following analysis examines whether citizens' involvement in political associations and participation in accountability actions enhance the effectiveness of health development interventions, controlling for the same set of socioeconomic and sociopolitical variables as in the previous section. The findings are detailed in the table below.

Table 5.2 reports the estimated effects on infant mortality across different indicators of political engagement. The negative coefficient of health aid indicates that development assistance for health lowers infant mortality at mean levels of political engagement. Again, the interaction term is negative and statistically significant (except for Model 5), implying that health aid reduces infant mortality more effectively in more politically engaged societies. This result holds even after accounting for various alternative factors, including public-sector corruption, health workers density, and female education levels.[4]

Moreover, the observed synergistic interaction effect remains consistent across various political-engagement measures, including expert ratings and public-opinion data. For instance, in Models 1–2, political involvement is measured by the Civil Society Participation index. The results suggest that as civil-society organizations exert more political influence, health aid's impact on population health in recipient countries becomes more pronounced. This finding is replicated for different model specifications and alternative indicators of political involvement, including the Political and Professional Engagement index, which directly captures the share of citizens active in political associations and trade unions.

Looking at the extent to which civil-society organizations hold governments accountable provides additional evidence for the enhancing effect of political involvement (Models 5–6). Although the interaction coefficient fails to achieve conventional levels of statistical significance, the signs of the estimated coefficients all point to a synergistic relationship between civil society's demand for accountability and health aid.[5] In Models 7–8, using self-reported membership in political and professional associations as a measure of political involvement further supports the finding that political engagement makes aid work better. The GMM estimates for the WVS sample of recipient countries show a highly significant negative interaction term cross-validating the finding that higher levels of political engagement enhance the effectiveness of health aid.

To facilitate interpretation, figure 5.2 visualizes the estimated effects of health aid on infant mortality across observed levels of political engagement, as detailed in table 5.2. Precisely, the figure displays the marginal

Table 5.2. Political Engagement, Health Aid, and Population Health

	Dependent Variable: Infant Mortality Rate (Log Scale)							
	Civil Society Participation		Political and Professional Engagement		Diagonal Accountability		Membership in Political and Professional Associations	
	(1)	(2)	(3)	(4)	(5)	(6)	(7)	(8)
DAH (log scale)	−0.025**	−0.026***	−0.013*	−0.011	−0.025**	−0.024**	−0.023	−0.039**
	(0.010)	(0.010)	(0.008)	(0.008)	(0.012)	(0.010)	(0.049)	(0.016)
Political engagement	−0.057	−0.038	0.012	0.009	0.006	0.008	0.153	0.113
	(0.087)	(0.092)	(0.027)	(0.020)	(0.030)	(0.027)	(0.428)	(0.243)
DAH (log scale) * Political engagement	−0.079**	−0.076***	−0.014*	−0.012**	−0.016	−0.013*	−0.361***	−0.378***
	(0.033)	(0.026)	(0.008)	(0.006)	(0.010)	(0.007)	(0.090)	(0.119)
Public-sector corruption control	0.044	0.058	−0.119	−0.123	−0.020	−0.024	−0.061	0.008
	(0.121)	(0.111)	(0.118)	(0.120)	(0.118)	(0.111)	(0.257)	(0.135)
IMR (lagged)	1.115***	1.119***	1.147***	1.090***	1.149***	1.126***	0.886***	0.822***
	(0.059)	(0.053)	(0.068)	(0.054)	(0.058)	(0.057)	(0.175)	(0.106)
Constant	0.000	−0.871*	0.000	0.000	−0.870**	0.000	0.000	0.000
	(0.000)	(0.504)	(0.000)	(0.000)	(0.383)	(0.000)	(0.000)	(0.000)
Conflict	Yes	Yes	Yes	Yes	Yes	Yes	Yes	Yes
GDP per capita (log scale)	Yes	Yes	Yes	Yes	Yes	Yes	Yes	Yes

	Dependent Variable: Infant Mortality Rate (Log Scale)							
	Civil Society Participation		Political and Professional Engagement		Diagonal Accountability		Membership in Political and Professional Associations	
	(1)	(2)	(3)	(4)	(5)	(6)	(7)	(8)
Population (log scale)	Yes	Yes	Yes	Yes	Yes	Yes	Yes	Yes
Fertility rate (log scale)		Yes		Yes		Yes		Yes
Physicians (log scale)	Yes	Yes	Yes	Yes	Yes	Yes	Yes	Yes
Female education (log scale)	Yes	Yes	Yes	Yes	Yes	Yes	Yes	Yes
Period FE	Yes	Yes	Yes	Yes	Yes	Yes	Yes	Yes
Observations	342	342	277	277	342	342	89	89
Countries	101	101	83	83	101	101	51	51
Instruments	77	86	77	86	77	86	37	40
Hansen-test	0.231	0.284	0.372	0.494	0.152	0.266	0.269	0.241
AR2	0.119	0.115	0.767	0.937	0.091	0.098		

Note: Table shows two-step GMM estimation with Windmeijer bias-corrected robust standard errors. Health aid (DAH) is lagged by one period. Political engagement is measured by the Civil Society Participation index (Models 1–2), Political and Professional Engagement index (Models 3–4), Diagonal Accountability index (Models 5–6), and the Membership in Political and Professional Associations index (Models 7–8). DAH and political engagement are mean-centered. *** $p < 0.01$, ** $p < 0.05$, * $p < 0.1$.

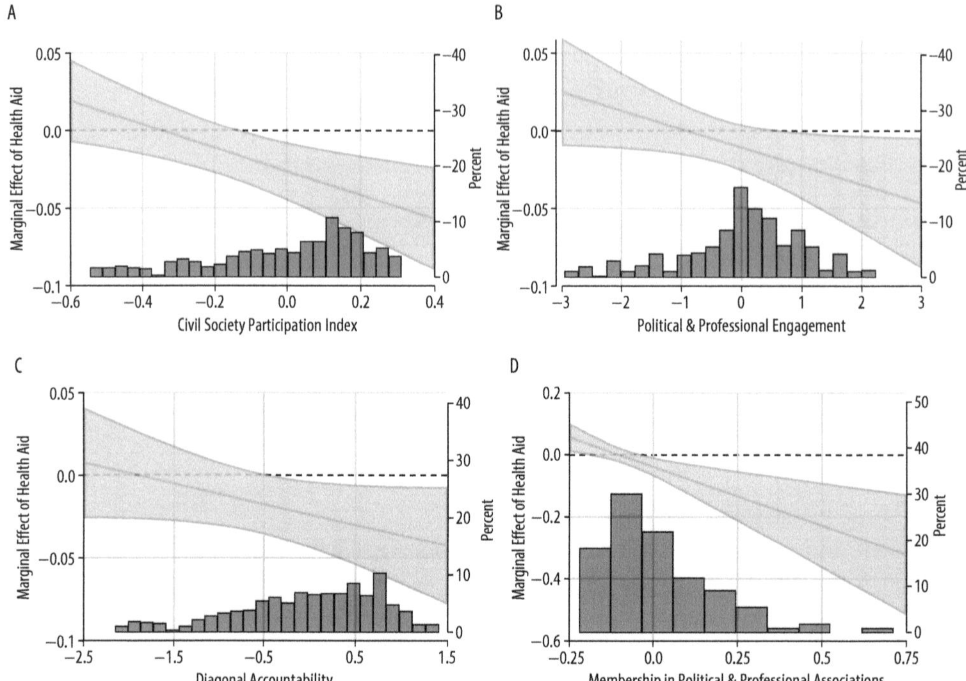

Figure 5.2. Political Engagement and the Marginal Effect of Health Aid. *Note:* Figure shows the average marginal effects of lagged health aid on infant mortality (with 95 percent confidence interval) based on two-step system-GMM estimations for different measures of political engagement. Each plot visualizes the estimated effects of lagged health aid across observed levels of (A) the Civil Society Participation index, (B) the Political and Professional Engagement index, (C) the Diagonal Accountability index, as well as (D) membership in political and professional associations. Estimates are based on Models 2, 4, 6, and 8 reported in table 5.2.

effect of lagged health aid across observed levels of (A) civil-society participation, (B) political and professional engagement, (C) diagonal accountability, and (D) citizens' self-reported membership in political and professional associations. Each plot demonstrates that the marginal effect of health aid in countries with a politically inactive citizenry is insignificant. Conversely, health aid has a significantly negative effect on infant mortality in countries with higher levels of political engagement.

The parameter estimates of Models 1–2 suggest that health aid significantly lowers infant mortality at levels of political engagement greater than the bottom 30 percent of the distribution. For example, in a country where civil-society organizations effectively translate their activism into political influence, like Nigeria in the late 1990s after transitioning from military rule, doubling health aid would reduce infant mortality by about 4.3 percent.[6] By contrast, in a country with moderately politically active citizens, the decline would amount to about 2.6 percent, all other factors being equal.

For countries surveyed by the WVS, the estimated effect of involvement in political associations is even larger (figure 5.2D). Specifically, in countries with highly politically active citizens (+1 standard deviation), doubling health aid per capita would reduce infant mortality by about 10.4 percent. Such a level of political engagement is similar to the situation in Albania in the late 1990s, where several large-scale trade unions, international and domestic NGOs, and political parties were competing for political influence despite minor government restrictions and regional instability resulting from the Kosovo conflict (Karatnycky 2000, 42–44). These findings imply that political engagement can make a vital contribution to increase health aid effectiveness.

In sum, the results show that the larger civil societies' capacity to transform activism into political influence, the larger the negative effect of lagged health aid on infant mortality. This finding supports Hypothesis 1b. Comparing the impact of doubling health aid between countries with moderately and highly politically active citizenries suggests that a one standard deviation increase in the share of politically involved citizens would increase the impact of health aid on declines in infant mortality by factor 1.5 and 2.5, respectively. In other words, the effectiveness of health aid increases when governments are held accountable by a politically engaged citizenry. The next section will delve into the specific role of mass action for accountability by examining the effects of citizen participation in elite-challenging activities.

Table 5.3 documents the interaction of health aid with citizens' engagement in elite-challenging actions, including pro-democratic mass events and anti-system movements. Controlling for other socioeconomic and sociopolitical determinants of public health, the interaction coefficient is significantly negative across all models. The test statistics further suggest that the endogeneity of aid is properly addressed. These results imply that health aid is more effective in countries where citizen participation in democratic mass movements or anti-system movements is more prevalent.

Table 5.3. Elite-Challenging Action, Health Aid, and Population Health

	Dependent Variable: Infant Mortality Rate (Log Scale)			
	Pro-Democratic Movements		Anti-System Movements	
	(1)	(2)	(3)	(4)
DAH (log scale)	−0.009	−0.009	−0.021**	−0.022***
	(0.010)	(0.010)	(0.010)	(0.008)
Elite-challenging action	0.029*	0.029	0.027	0.030*
	(0.015)	(0.018)	(0.018)	(0.018)
DAH (log scale) * Elite-challenging action	−0.015**	−0.017**	−0.019**	−0.021***
	(0.007)	(0.007)	(0.009)	(0.008)
Public-sector corruption control	−0.083	0.043	−0.079	−0.025
	(0.086)	(0.121)	(0.112)	(0.119)
Government health expenditures		−0.009*		−0.005
		(0.005)		(0.004)
IMR (lagged)	1.044***	1.030***	0.995***	1.006***
	(0.053)	(0.055)	(0.050)	(0.051)
Constant	−0.151	0.000	0.000	0.135
	(0.380)	(0.000)	(0.000)	(0.389)
Population (log scale)	Yes	Yes	Yes	Yes
Conflict	Yes	Yes	Yes	Yes
GDP per capita (log scale)	Yes	Yes	Yes	Yes
HIV prevalence (log scale)	Yes	Yes	Yes	Yes
Period FE	Yes	Yes	Yes	Yes
Observations	324	320	422	418
Countries	86	85	109	108
Instruments	71	76	71	76
Hansen-test	0.192	0.174	0.099	0.095
AR2	0.742	0.935	0.296	0.196

Note: Table shows two-step GMM estimation with Windmeijer bias-corrected robust standard errors. Elite-challenging action is measured by the Pro-Democratic Movements index (Models 1–2) and the Anti-System Movements index (Models 3–4). Health aid (DAH) is lagged by one period. Both DAH and elite-challenging action are mean-centered.
*** $p < 0.01$, ** $p < 0.05$, * $p < 0.1$.

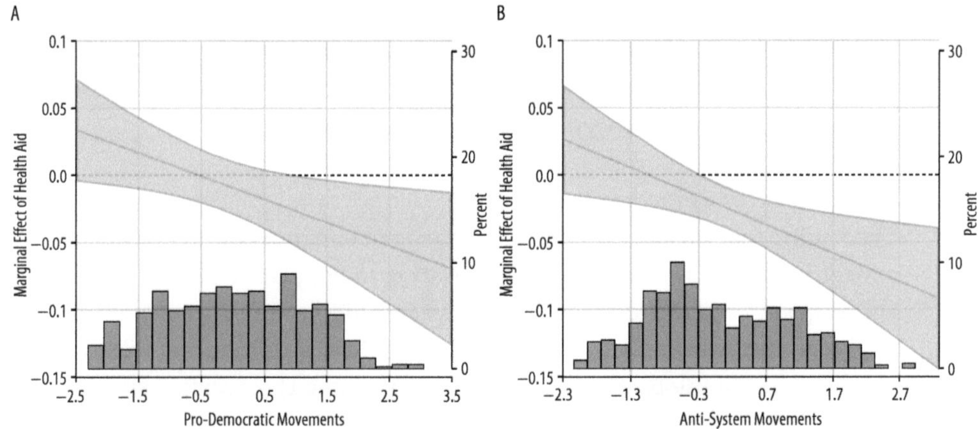

Figure 5.3. Elite-Challenging Action and the Marginal Effect of Health Aid. *Note:* Figure shows the average marginal effects of lagged health aid on infant mortality (with 95 percent confidence interval) based on two-step system-GMM estimations for different measures of elite-challenging mass movements. Each plot visualizes the estimated effects of lagged health aid across observed levels of (A) pro-democratic mass events and (B) anti-system opposition movements. Estimates are based on Model 2 and Model 4 reported in table 5.3.

Supplementary evidence supports the robustness of these findings (as detailed in table A5.5 and table A5.6). In sum, elite-challenging actions can improve the effectiveness of health aid, regardless of whether participants seek to protect and advance democratic rights or are more ideologically oriented and aim to change the polity in fundamental ways.

Figure 5.3 visualizes the estimated effects of lagged health aid on infant mortality across observed levels of (A) pro-democratic mass events and (B) anti-system oppositional movements. The figure shows that higher levels of both pro-democratic and anti-system actions are associated with a stronger negative effect of aid, implying that elite-challenging actions enhance the effectiveness of health aid. For example, in a country like Jordan in the early 2010s, where a considerable number of popular mass movements sought to advance democratic rights and demanded political reforms, doubling health aid would reduce infant mortality by about 3 percent. While anti-system oppositional movements show similar effects, the impact is slightly more pronounced for pro-democratic movements.[7] Specifically, a one standard deviation increase in citizens' participation in elite-challenging activities could more than double the decline in infant mortality resulting from health aid. These results lend support to Hypothesis 1c, which states that elite-challenging political engagement makes aid work better.

Accounting for Selection Bias

The finding that social and political engagement enhances the effectiveness of health aid is based on examining variation in population health among aid recipients. Countries that did not receive aid have been omitted. By solely concentrating on aid recipients, there is the risk of inducing selectivity bias because unobserved factors that determine the sample selection are likely to be correlated with the dependent variable (Heckman 1979). Specifically, previous research has shown that a large share of health aid is allocated to fragile, unstable (low- and middle-income) countries with high corruption and weak state capacity (Graves, Haakenstad, and Dieleman 2015, 1). Thus, we expect that the unobserved factors determining whether a country receives health aid are correlated with the unobserved factors determining infant mortality.

To ensure unbiased estimates, the following section replicates the previous analyses on the determinants of public health using a Heckman two-stage selection model, in particular, a random-effects linear regression model with endogenous sample selection.[8] The Heckman approach includes a first-stage probit model that captures why some countries are more likely to receive health aid (DAH recipient equation) based on the most important determinants, including a country's level of economic development and corruption control, as well as the quality of health infrastructure and democratic institutions. This information is then used in the second-stage regression, which computes the effect of health aid on infant mortality (IMR equation).

The results of the Heckman model confirm the previously identified synergistic interaction between lagged health aid and civic engagement across various model specifications, as detailed in table A5.7–table A5.9.[9] The negative sign of the coefficient of health aid (in the IMR equation) indicates a mortality-reducing effect of development assistance for health (at mean levels of social or political engagement). And the significant interaction term replicates the identified synergistic relationship in which both civic engagement and health aid per capita improve population health. As these results are robust to the inclusion of various control variables, this finding implies that health aid per capita is more effective in reducing infant mortality in countries with higher social and political engagement levels after accounting for endogenous sample selection.

The size of the estimated enhancing effect of civic engagement after accounting for selectivity bias is similar to previous estimates. Likewise, the positive correlation between the panel-level random effect for the IMR and the selection model suggests that unobserved observation-level factors that increase the chance of being a health aid recipient tend to increase countries' infant mortality rates. These results provide additional evidence of an enhancing interaction pattern between development assistance for health and civic engagement, accounting for the tendency of countries that are less likely to advance population health to receive aid.

Civic Engagement vs. Top-Down Mechanisms of Performance Oversight

Previous aid effectiveness studies have largely ignored citizen demand for accountability and focused on formally institutionalized accountability mechanisms, particularly those associated with higher state capacity and liberal democracy. This focus has failed to provide conclusive evidence regarding the role of context conditions that make aid more effective. Against this backdrop, the following section examines the role of countries' formal political context—including state capacity and democracy—compared to the role of citizen engagement. Specifying bottom-up and top-down accountability mechanisms as moderators of health aid in the same model allows for directly comparing each mechanism's relevance. Moreover, this approach serves as a robustness check, strengthening the validity of the civic engagement hypothesis.

State capacity is reflected by the quality of bureaucratic governance and is measured by different indicators, including the Quality of Government and the State Fragility indices. Supplementary analyses test the robustness of the results using several additional indicators of corruption control, including control over regime, executive, and public-sector corruption. Each replication model tests whether the effect of health aid on population health is moderated by state capacity while applying the same model specifications and accounting for the same set of control variables as before.

The results reported in tables A5.10 and A5.11 of the appendix demonstrate that the effectiveness of health aid does not significantly differ across countries with varying levels of state capacity. In none of the models did health aid and bureaucratic governance interact significantly. In other words, there is no indication the effect of health aid varies across different levels of states' capacity to manage conflict, make and implement public policy, and deliver essential services once we account for the conditioning role of civic engagement. Instead, testing the interaction of health aid with civic engagement and state capacity simultaneously demonstrates it is primarily civic engagement that makes health aid work better. This is indicated by the significant interaction between health aid and social engagement and the insignificant interaction between health aid and bureaucratic governance across different model specifications and measures of state capacity, as detailed in table A5.12.[10] Comparing the role of state capacity with political instead of social engagement leads to qualitatively similar results.

The aid effectiveness literature has also examined the moderating role of democratic institutions. For instance, Svensson (1999) provides evidence that political rights and civil liberties enhance the effects of aggregate aid on economic growth, arguing that democratic governments are more accountable for the way foreign aid is spent. Hence, to compare the conditioning role of democratic institutions with the identified effects of civic engagement, the next section delves into the interactions between health aid and democratic institutions that capture the extent of judicial and legislative constraints, executive oversight, and the extent of horizontal and overall accountability. I also use three composite democracy indices to operationalize the concept of democracy more broadly, including the Polity IV index, the Freedom House index, and the Coalition to Selectorate Size ratio.[11] To test the interaction of health aid with civic engagement and democratic institutions simultaneously, each model accounts for the same set of control variables and applies the same model specification as before.

Comparing both moderating effects demonstrates the importance of citizen engagement over institutionalized oversight mechanisms. The GMM estimates reported in table A5.13 in the appendix show that health aid significantly interacts with social engagement but not with any of the top-down measures of democratic oversight. Again, using political instead of social engagement leads to qualitatively similar results. These results demonstrate that differences in health aid effectiveness do not primarily result from variations in countries' legislative or judicial oversight over the executive, aggregate levels of (horizontal) accountability, or the overall quality of liberal democracy. Instead, it is citizens' associational involvement that makes health aid work better. Hence, while there is no indication that the effect of health aid varies across different levels of institutionalized performance oversight, the evidence suggests that increased citizen participation in bottom-up processes of performance oversight makes health aid more effective.

Individual Well-Being and Aid Effectiveness: A Multilevel Perspective

The previous analysis has shown that civic engagement enhances the effects of aid on public health at the country level. By implication, we would expect citizen participation also to impact the effects of aid on individuals' health. Therefore, the enhancing effects of social and political engagement should be observable at the country level and when analyzing individual health outcomes. The following section applies standard linear multilevel regression analysis to test the proposed synergistic interaction between health aid and civic engagement on individuals' health status. The multilevel approach accounts for the clustered data structure and eliminates differences linked to country-specific features of the sociopolitical and socioeconomic context.[12]

To investigate whether civic engagement enhances the effects of health aid on individuals' health status, the next section analyzes data from 50 countries, covering about 100,000 individuals over the period 1995–2015.[13] Individuals' self-reported health status is measured on a 5-point scale, with ratings ranging from very poor to very good health, and is normalized to an index ranging from 0 to 1. Self-rated health is recognized as a valid measure of individuals' objective health status and has been extensively used in public-health research (Wu et al. 2013, 1). Numerous studies have confirmed the relationship between self-rated health and mortality, demonstrating that lower health ratings correspond with increased mortality risk (Jylhä 2009).[14]

A closer examination of the self-rated health data reveals that about 12 percent of the variation in beneficiaries' health status can be attributed to the distinct macro-level characteristics of recipient countries. To determine whether social and political engagement enhances aid effectiveness at the individual level, the multilevel analysis examines the interaction of civic engagement and health aid, using the same measures as in the previous analyses. Given the inverse correlation between self-rated health and mortality levels, a synergistic relationship between health aid and civic engagement is indicated if all three country-level coefficients show a positive sign. I further account for the quality of reproductive health care and countries' socioeconomic context, including factors like economic development, population size, conflict involvement, and public-sector corruption. Additionally, the model accounts for the prevalence of HIV/AIDS, female fertility rates, and governments' domestic health expenditures. To mitigate potential bias from unobserved factors of population health, the multilevel models also include period-fixed effects.

At the individual level, all models control for respondents' age, sex, income, and education, addressing differences in self-rated health among beneficiaries with different socioeconomic backgrounds. Additional individual-level control variables include respondents' satisfaction with life and interest in politics, as well as individuals' membership in voluntary associations.[15] It is worth noting that while the direct effects of social engagement on individual well-being are well documented in public-health and social-capital research, the focus of this analysis lies on the moderating effect of aggregate levels of citizen involvement.[16] To facilitate interpretation, income, life satisfaction, and political interest are rescaled into a range from 0 to 1. Likewise, following standard practice, all individual-level variables are centered on their group mean, and country-level variables are centered on their respective global mean.

Table 5.4 reports the results of the multilevel linear regression with country random intercepts and shows the estimated effects of civic engagement and health aid on individuals' self-reported health status. The positive coefficients of aggregate civic engagement and DAH indicate that both citizen involvement and development assistance for health (at mean levels of each other) improve individual health in recipient countries. Notably, adding the interaction of civic engagement and health aid further improves the model fit, as indicated by the reported AIC and BIC values (Baguley 2012, 402). The significant positive interaction term implies that citizen participation further enhances the positive effects of health aid on self-rated health, confirming the proposed enhancing effect of civic engagement after accounting for the nested data structure. The identified synergistic interaction pattern remains robust when controlling for various individual and country-level covariates, including public-sector corruption. Likewise, the controls show the expected signs indicating that individual income, political interest, and life

Table 5.4. Civic Engagement, Health Aid, and Individual Health

	Dependent Variable: Self-Rated Health Status				
	(1)	(2)	(3)	(4)	(5)
Country Level					
DAH (log scale)	−0.000	0.001	0.001**	0.002**	0.002***
	(0.001)	(0.001)	(0.001)	(0.001)	(0.001)
Civic engagement		0.05***	0.04***	0.05***	0.06***
		(0.013)	(0.013)	(0.011)	(0.011)
DAH (log scale) * Civic engagement			0.01***	0.01***	0.01***
			(0.003)	(0.003)	(0.003)
Public-sector corruption control	−0.006	−0.009	−0.06**	−0.07**	
	(0.027)	(0.026)	(0.029)	(0.029)	
Government health expenditures	−0.002***	−0.001*	−0.00		
	(0.001)	(0.001)	(0.001)		
Individual Level					
Income	0.075***	0.075***	0.07***	0.07***	0.07***
	(0.003)	(0.003)	(0.003)	(0.003)	(0.003)
Member in any voluntary association	0.006***	0.005***	0.01***	0.01***	0.01***
	(0.001)	(0.001)	(0.001)	(0.001)	(0.001)
Life satisfaction	0.192***	0.192***	0.19***	0.19***	0.19***
	(0.003)	(0.003)	(0.003)	(0.002)	(0.002)
Political interest	0.011***	0.011***	0.01***	0.01***	0.01***
	(0.002)	(0.002)	(0.002)	(0.002)	(0.002)
Constant	0.084	0.102	0.17	0.15	0.02
	(0.196)	(0.182)	(0.177)	(0.171)	(0.175)
Country-Level Controls					
Period FE	Yes	Yes	Yes	Yes	Yes
Conflict	Yes	Yes	Yes	Yes	Yes
Population (log scale)	Yes	Yes	Yes	Yes	Yes
GDP per capita (log scale)	Yes	Yes	Yes	Yes	Yes
Fertility rate (log scale)	Yes	Yes	Yes	Yes	Yes
Individual-Level Controls					
Education	Yes	Yes	Yes	Yes	Yes
Sex	Yes	Yes	Yes	Yes	Yes
Age	Yes	Yes	Yes	Yes	Yes

(continued)

Table 5.4. Civic Engagement, Health Aid, and Individual Health (continued)

	Dependent Variable: Self-Rated Health Status				
	(1)	(2)	(3)	(4)	(5)
Observations	94,130	94,130	94,130	95,622	95,622
Countries	49	49	49	50	50
chi2	7,528	7,392	7,407	7,653	7,649
ICC	0.38	0.34	0.32	0.34	0.31
AIC	−51,466	−51,479	−51,494	−52,286	−52,283
BIC	−51,277	−51,281	−51,286	−52,088	−52,094
Log likelihood	25,753	25,761	25,769	26,164	26,162

Note: Table shows estimates of multilevel linear regression with random intercept. Civic engagement at the country level is measured as the share of population belonging to any voluntary association using data from the WVS. DAH and civic engagement are global mean-centered. Standard errors in parentheses. *** $p < 0.01$, ** $p < 0.05$, * $p < 0.1$.
Source: WVS 1995–2015.

satisfaction are positively associated with health status. Similarly, individual associational membership has a significant positive effect on individual well-being, supporting previous evidence (Kawachi, Kennedy, Glass 1999; Helliwell and Putnam 2004; Kawachi, Subramanian, and Kim 2008).

To further examine whether there is a difference between social and political engagement, I estimate the effects of health aid and membership for leisure and welfare, political and professional, and faith-based associations separately. For each purpose of participation, I test the additive effects of lagged health aid and civic engagement (Model 1) as well as the interaction effects of health aid and citizen engagement after accounting for conflict involvement, population size, GDP per capita, and female fertility (Model 2), public-sector corruption control (Model 3), and government health expenditures (Model 4).

Table 5.5 summarizes the main results of the multilevel analyses. Concerning engagement in leisure and welfare organizations, the reported estimates suggest that a larger share of citizen involvement fosters the positive effect of aid on individuals' self-reported health status (panel 1). This effect is robust to the inclusion of various controls. The effect of civic engagement is strongest, however, in politically engaged societies. In particular, membership in political parties, labor unions, and professional organizations has the largest impact on enhancing the effectiveness of

	Dependent Variable: Self-Rated Health Status			
	(1)	(2)	(3)	(4)
Panel 1				
DAH (log scale)	0.003***	0.00***	0.00***	0.00***
	(0.001)	(0.001)	(0.001)	(0.001)
Engagement in leisure and welfare associations	0.105***	0.113***	0.113***	0.106***
	(0.013)	(0.012)	(0.012)	(0.013)
DAH (log scale) * Engagement in leisure and welfare associations		0.01**	0.01**	0.01
		(0.003)	(0.004)	(0.004)
Panel 2				
DAH (log scale)	0.001*	0.01***	0.01***	0.01***
	(0.001)	(0.001)	(0.001)	(0.001)
Engagement in political and professional associations	0.162***	0.22***	0.22***	0.21***
	(0.014)	(0.015)	(0.015)	(0.015)
DAH (log scale) * Engagement in political and professional associations		0.07***	0.07***	0.07***
		(0.005)	(0.005)	(0.005)
Panel 3				
DAH (log scale)	0.001*	0.00*	0.00***	0.00**
	(0.001)	(0.001)	(0.001)	(0.001)
Engagement in faith-based associations	−0.030***	−0.00	0.00	−0.026**
	(0.011)	(0.009)	(0.009)	(0.011)
DAH (log scale) * Engagement in faith-based associations		−0.015***	−0.022***	−0.021***
		(0.003)	(0.003)	(0.003)
Country-Level Controls				
Conflict	Yes	Yes	Yes	Yes
Population (log scale)	Yes	Yes	Yes	Yes
GDP per capita (log scale)	Yes	Yes	Yes	Yes
Fertility rate (log scale)	Yes	Yes	Yes	Yes
Public-sector corruption control	Yes		Yes	Yes
Government health expenditures	Yes			Yes
Period FE	Yes	Yes	Yes	Yes

Table 5.5. Social and Political Engagement, Health Aid, and Individual Health (continued)

	Dependent Variable: Self-Rated Health Status			
	(1)	(2)	(3)	(4)
Individual-Level Controls				
Education	Yes	Yes	Yes	Yes
Income	Yes	Yes	Yes	Yes
Life satisfaction	Yes	Yes	Yes	Yes
Political interest	Yes	Yes	Yes	Yes
Sex	Yes	Yes	Yes	Yes
Age	Yes	Yes	Yes	Yes
Member in any voluntary association	Yes	Yes	Yes	Yes
N	≥ 92,901	≥ 94,393	≥ 94,393	≥ 92,901
Countries	49	50	50	49

Note: Table shows estimates of multilevel linear regression with random intercept including the main and interaction effects of health aid with the share of population belonging to leisure and welfare organizations (panel 1), faith-based associations (panel 2), and political and professional organizations (panel 3). DAH and civic-engagement variables are global mean-centered. Standard errors in parentheses. *** $p < 0.01$, ** $p < 0.05$, * $p < 0.1$.
Source: WVS 1995–2015.

health aid (panel 2). These results differ from citizen involvement in religious organizations. The reported estimates suggest that a larger percentage of citizens engaging in faith-based organizations weakens the effects of development assistance on individual health (panel 3).[17] This result aligns with findings from chapter 4, which indicate that members of faith-based organizations are less supportive of liberal democracy and civic values. It also echoes with the finding that memberships in "isolated" associations (including faith-based organizations) create less trust than involvement in "connected" associations whose members have many ties to other associations and thus "are more likely to cross-cut social boundaries and promote contact with diverse others" (Paxton 2007, 56).

The multilevel analyses reported in table 5.5 demonstrate that elite-entrusting forms of political engagement and citizen involvement in leisure and welfare associations strengthen the positive effect of health aid on individuals' self-rated health status, whereas religious engagement weakens health aid effectiveness. Given that political engagement also involves social-movement activities, especially where formal avenues of political participation are limited (Harris and Hern 2018, 11), it is worth exploring the role of elite-challenging activities. The results on the role of elite-challenging accountability actions are reported in table 5.6, corroborating the importance of citizen engagement. Specifically, the reported estimates add further evidence that health aid improves individual health in countries with an active citizenry willing and able to exercise pressure through citizen-led accountability actions, including protests.[18]

To gain clearer insights into the identified relationships, figure 5.4 visualizes the estimated interaction patterns between health aid and civic engagement. The figure displays the marginal effect of lagged health aid on self-rated health across observed levels of citizens' participation in leisure and welfare organizations (A), political and professional organizations (B), faith-based associations (C), and elite-challenging action (D). The different plots demonstrate how the moderating effects of social and political engagement on self-reported health vary by the specific type of engagement.

The plot (B) indicates a strong synergistic interaction pattern for political engagement. Specifically, as the share of citizens involved in political parties, labor unions, or professional organizations increases, the positive effect of health aid on individual health becomes more pronounced. To illustrate, doubling health aid in a recipient country with a highly politically active citizenry one standard deviation above the mean would increase individuals' health ratings by about one point on a 5-point scale of self-rated health. When considering engagement in leisure and welfare organizations (A), there is also a synergistic interaction pattern, but the magnitude of the moderating effect is modest. In contrast, for citizen engagement in faith-based associations (C), the effect is reverse, implying that in countries with a significant share of the population engaged in faith-based organizations, an increase in health aid might harm rather than improve individual health.

Plot (D) shows that elite-challenging actions may either strengthen the positive effect of health aid on individual health or make ineffective aid less harmful. To clarify, in recipient countries where citizens are either not used to or prevented from demanding accountability through protests, increasing aid adversely affects individual health.[19] Yet, across countries with rising levels of elite-challenging action, the adverse effects of health aid decrease and ultimately disappear. In fact, as protest levels rise above

Table 5.6. Elite-Challenging Action, Health Aid, and Individual Health

	Dependent Variable: Self-Rated Health Status				
	(1)	(2)	(3)	(4)	(5)
Country Level					
DAH (log scale)	−0.001	−0.002***	−0.000	−0.001	−0.000
	(0.001)	(0.001)	(0.001)	(0.001)	(0.001)
Elite-challenging action	0.066*	0.029	0.124***	0.067	0.044
	(0.034)	(0.035)	(0.040)	(0.042)	(0.041)
DAH (log scale) * Elite-challenging action	0.077***	0.115***	0.125***	0.144***	0.113***
	(0.014)	(0.014)	(0.015)	(0.016)	(0.016)
Individual Level					
Income	0.072***	0.117***	0.122***	0.121***	0.075***
	(0.003)	(0.003)	(0.003)	(0.003)	(0.003)
Elite-challenging action	0.002	−0.006**	0.003	−0.002	0.004
	(0.003)	(0.003)	(0.003)	(0.004)	(0.003)
Member in voluntary association	0.004**	0.008***	0.009***	0.008***	0.004**
	(0.002)	(0.002)	(0.002)	(0.002)	(0.002)
Life satisfaction	0.189***				0.184***
	(0.003)				(0.003)
Political interest	0.011***	0.015***		0.018***	0.014***
	(0.002)	(0.002)		(0.003)	(0.002)
Constant	0.369**	0.532***	−0.123	0.056	−0.098
	(0.180)	(0.152)	(0.209)	(0.216)	(0.241)
Country-Level Controls					
Period FE	Yes	Yes	Yes	Yes	Yes
Conflict	Yes	Yes	Yes	Yes	Yes
Government health expenditures	Yes	Yes		Yes	Yes
Public-sector corruption control	Yes	Yes	Yes	Yes	Yes
Fertility rate (log scale)	Yes	Yes	Yes	Yes	Yes
HIV prevalence (log scale)			Yes	Yes	Yes
Population (log scale)	Yes	Yes	Yes	Yes	Yes
GDP per capita (log scale)	Yes	Yes	Yes	Yes	Yes
Individual-Level Controls					
Education	Yes	Yes	Yes	Yes	Yes
Sex	Yes	Yes	Yes	Yes	Yes
Age	Yes	Yes	Yes	Yes	Yes

	Dependent Variable: Self-Rated Health Status				
	(1)	(2)	(3)	(4)	(5)
Observations	80,610	81,067	62,632	60,718	60,378
Countries	45	45	33	32	32
chi2	6,220	5,688	3,904	3,535	4,018
ICC	0.31	0.22	0.30	0.31	0.39
AIC	−44,631	−40,107	−32,375	−31,520	−34,621
BIC	−44,418	−39,903	−32,185	−31,312	−34,405
Log likelihood	22,339	20,076	16,208	15,783	17,335

Note: Table shows estimates of multilevel linear regression with random intercept. Elite-challenging action is measured by the Social Movement Activity index. DAH and elite-challenging action are global mean-centered. Standard errors in parentheses.
Source: WVS 1995–2015. *** $p < 0.01$, ** $p < 0.05$, * $p < 0.1$.

average, the figure shows that the more citizens are involved, the more aid works. Yet the magnitude of this effect on individual health is relatively small compared to the enhancing effect of citizens' participation in political and professional organizations. In other words, citizen-led accountability action makes aid work better either by buffering the adverse effects of ineffective aid practices or enhancing the effectiveness of health aid.

Summary

To summarize, this chapter presents compelling evidence that social and political engagement significantly enhances the impact of aid on population and individual health as citizens involved in outward-oriented social networks and those participating in political associations and accountability actions are better positioned and motivated to engage in development projects affecting their communities and to hold authorities to account.

A panel study has shown that both social engagement and political engagement substantially enhance the negative effects of health aid on infant mortality levels. The synergistic relationship implies that development assistance for health more effectively improves population health in recipient countries where citizens regularly attend community meetings, engage in voluntary associations, and actively participate in elite-challenging political activities.

This result builds upon the finding that citizens in vibrant societies are more interested in community matters, share civic values, and are likely to

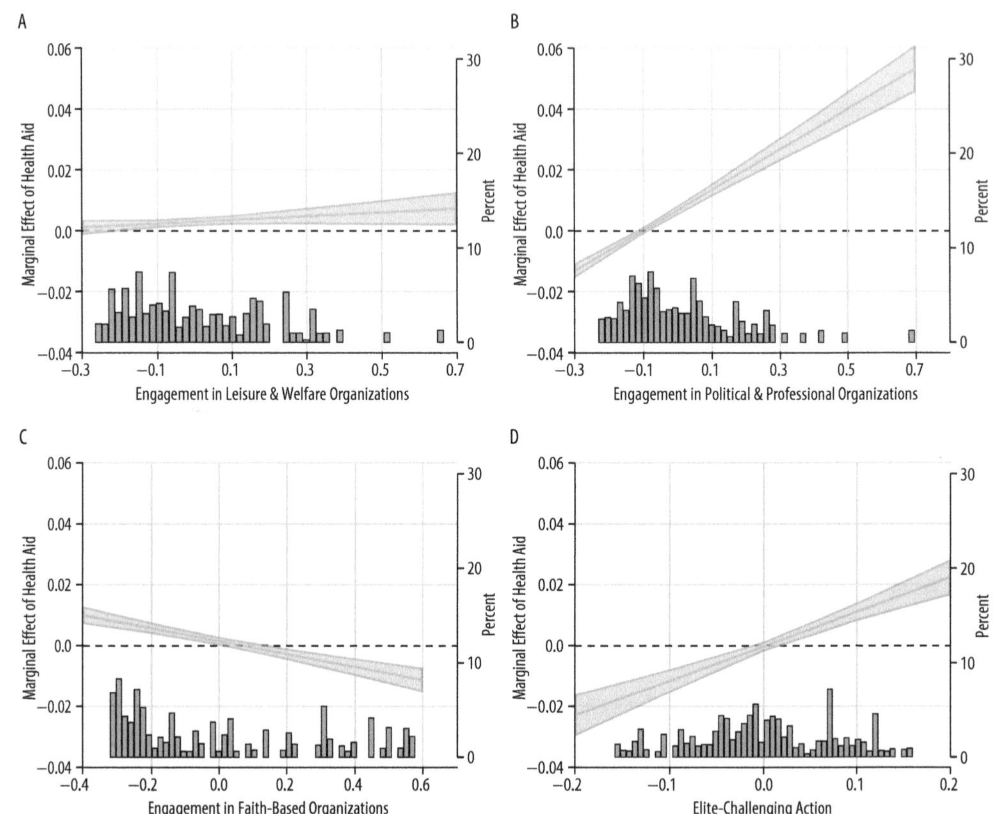

Figure 5.4. Civic Engagement and the Marginal Effect of Health Aid on Individual Health. *Note:* The figure shows the average marginal effects of lagged health aid on individuals' self-reported health status at varying levels of citizen engagement in leisure and welfare organizations (A), political and professional organizations (B), faith-based associations (C), and elite-challenging action (D) (with 95 percent confidence intervals). Estimates are reported in table 5.5 (Model 4, panels 1–3) and table 5.6 (Model 5).

cooperate and engage in accountability actions. Given that active citizenries are more willing and capable to voice shared concerns and exercise pressure on public authorities, the observed synergistic relationship implies that citizens' demand for accountability increases the effectiveness of health aid.

The results are consistent across different indicators of social and political engagement while accounting for simultaneity bias and endogenous sample selection. Comparing the effects of citizen-led accountability mechanisms with formally institutionalized oversight mechanisms further reveals that citizen engagement, rather than formal political institutions, matters the most. In particular, once civic engagement is taken into account, neither state capacity nor democratic institutions play a determining role in the effectiveness of health aid.

The evidence suggests that strengthening social and, in particular, political engagement has a large potential to improve public health. Estimates suggest that the presence of a diverse set of civil-society organizations that have the capacity to hold governments accountable and translate activism into political influence would, on average, double health aid's effect on declines in infant mortality. For citizens' participation in elite-challenging action—particularly those that seek to protect and advance democratic rights—the estimated gains in aid effectiveness are even larger.

A multilevel study further shows that civic engagement also strengthens the positive impact of aid on individual well-being. Specifically, political engagement and involvement in leisure and welfare associations enhance the benefits of health aid on individuals' self-rated health. Political and professional organizations show the strongest effect. This enhancing effect is not observed for faith-based organizations, however, whose members put less emphasis on voice and accountability.

Overall, the reported evidence demonstrates that socially and politically active communities can make aid improve population health and individual well-being. To further examine the supply-side conditions under which social and political engagement enhance health aid effectiveness, the following section inspects whether the combined effect of civic engagement and health aid varies across different institutional contexts.

NOTES

1. Using the estimates displayed in figure 5.1B, doubling health aid in a country where many citizens are active in independent non-political associations—as observed in Botswana in the early 2010s, where citizens enjoyed a relatively high level of interpersonal trust and cooperation—would reduce infant mortality by about 3.5 percent, compared to a 1.7 percent decline in countries with a moderately active citizenry. The estimated size of the enhancing effect based on the Social Engagement Index (figure 5.1D) is similar to the estimated difference between environments with moderate and high CSO involvement. At mean levels of citizens' participation in voluntary activities and community work, doubling health aid per capita would reduce infant mortality by about 2.7 percent and about 5.3 percent at high levels of citizen participation (one standard deviation above the mean). Paraguay and Nicaragua in the early 2010s represent typical

cases of moderate and high levels of civic involvement. In Paraguay, many citizens were involved in small-scale community organizations, although a general civic culture was absent, as the main objective for organizing was usually limited to immediate measures (BTI 2014). Similarly, in Nicaragua, many citizens were involved in informal self-help networks and social movements, including feminist and civil-liberties movements.

2. Table A5.1 and table A5.2 provide further evidence of the robustness of the findings after accounting for different sets of control variables and using a different estimation approach (LDV model).

3. Controlling for a country's membership in international NGOs or women's international NGOs leads to qualitatively similar results and adds further validity to the reported findings. While the effect of INGO connectedness on infant mortality is positive, it is mostly statistically insignificant and does not alter the interaction pattern between health aid and civic engagement. Similarly, a country's membership in WINGOs is found to be positively associated with infant mortality. But it largely lacks statistical significance and does not modify the relationship between health aid and civic engagement. Given that public health might affect the presence of international NGOs and women's international NGOs in recipient countries, each control is specified as an endogenous variable. Robustness results on INGO connectedness and WINGO memberships can be shared upon request.

4. Table A5.3 and table A5.4 document additional tests of robustness demonstrating that the capacity of civil-society organizations to translate activism into political influence and hold governments accountable makes health aid more effective.

5. Furthermore, testing the robustness of the identified interaction between health aid and diagonal accountability, table A5.4 confirms that health aid is more effective in reducing infant mortality when governments are held accountable through citizen-led accountability actions.

6. Using the estimates displayed in figure 5.2B, doubling health aid in a country where many citizens are active in independent political and professional associations—as observed in Cameroon in the early 2010s—would reduce infant mortality by about 2.4 percent, compared to about 1.1 percent in recipient countries with moderately active citizenries. The estimates based on the Diagonal Accountability index (figure 5.2C) suggest that if governments are held accountable by civil-society organizations, as observed in Hungary (one standard deviation above the mean) in the early 1990s, doubling health aid per capita would reduce infant mortality by about 3.4 percent.

7. For pro-democratic mass movements, doubling health aid is associated with a 1 percent decline in infant mortality in countries with moderate levels and a 3 percent decline in infant mortality in countries with high levels of elite-challenging actions. Conversely, for anti-system oppositional movements, the same effect amounts to about 2.2 percent in countries with moderate levels and about 4.6 percent in countries with high levels of anti-system movements.

8. Applying the standard Heckman two-stage selection models to panel data will provide inefficient estimates because it ignores the within-panel correlation. Instead, I use maximum likelihood estimation to model both the selection and outcome equations and account for the panel structure of the data using Stata's xtheckman command.

9. Civic engagement is measured by the Social Engagement Index (tables A5.7 and A5.8) and the Anti-System Movements index (table A5.9).

10. Only Model 2 indicates a marginally significant interaction effect between health aid and state capacity, although of opposite sign (table A5.12). This result suggests the effectiveness of health aid is higher in countries with less state capacity because state fragility is inversely coded and thus negatively correlated with state capacity, bureaucratic governance, and control of corruption.

11. Freedom House and Polity IV measure (each to a different extent) the existence of institutionalized constraints on the power of the executive, the presence of institutions and procedures through which citizens can express their preferences, and the guarantee of civil liberties to all citizens. The Coalition to Selectorate Size ratio is a measure of open and competitive executive recruitment and political participation that shape politicians' incentives for public-good provision.

12. Likelihood ratio tests indicate a better model fit of multilevel models compared to pooled linear models.

13. This period comprises three repeated cross-sectional samples from 1995–2000, 2005–2010, and 2010–2015. Data on citizen participation in voluntary associations in WVS Wave 4 (2000–2004) is unavailable.

14. Although this relationship seems universal, there is some evidence that relative differences exist between groups of different ages, sex, and socioeconomic backgrounds (Jylhä 2009).

15. Education is measured on a 3-point scale indicating individuals' highest educational level attained, ranging from lower to upper levels of education. Income is measured based on respondents' assessment of their household income on a 10-point scale, where 1 indicates the lowest income group and 10 the highest income group in each country. Age effects are captured based on respondents belonging to the following age groups: 15–24, 25–34, 35–44, 45–54, 55–64, or 65+. Life satisfaction is measured on a 10-point scale based on respondents' assessment of how satisfied they are with their lives as a whole. To measure political interest, I recode individuals' responses on their reported level of interest in politics into a 4-point scale ranging from "Not interested" (1) to "Very interested" (4).

16. In line with these findings, the multilevel analyses control for both individual associational membership and community social engagement (Kawachi, Kennedy, Glass 1999; Helliwell and Putnam 2004; Kawachi, Subramanian, and Kim 2008).

17. Tables A5.14–A5.16 of the appendix provide further evidence of the robustness of this finding.

18. Table A5.17 provides further evidence of the robustness of this finding.

19. In other words, if a recipient country receives above-average levels of health aid and has a politically inactive citizenry, individuals' predicted self-reported health status is lower than would be expected from the amount of health aid a country received alone. By contrast, if a recipient country receives above-average levels of health aid and has an above-average politically active citizenry, individuals' predicted self-reported health status is higher than would be expected from the amount of health aid a country received alone.

6

Civic Engagement in Varying Political Contexts

The previous analysis revealed that civic engagement enhances the positive effects of aid on public health. Although this finding underscores the importance of social and political engagement in making aid more effective, the specific political conditions maximizing this influence remain unclear. On the one hand, the extent to which the political context boosts citizen demand for accountability and government responsiveness is often cited to depend on states' capacity to allocate aid efficiently, the guarantee of political rights and civil liberties that protect citizens exercising voice, and the devolution of power and resources to subnational governments to respond to diverse local demands. On the other hand, citizen participation can increase government responsiveness even if a state lacks democratic oversight institutions (Gaventa and Barrett 2012) or administrative and organizational capacities (Risse, Börzel, and Draude 2018; Murtazashvili 2016). Strong institutions might even undermine the enhancing effects of civic engagement, for instance, if power-sharing arrangements between central and local authorities create incentives for corruption (Bardhan and Mookherjee 2006; Bardhan 2002).

Consequently, the following chapter systematically examines the institutional conditions under which civic engagement makes health aid work best and explores to what extent the enhancing impact of civic engagement is influenced by recipient countries' political context, including levels of bureaucratic governance, liberal democracy, and decentralization. The chapter answers this question by examining the three-way interactions between civic engagement, health aid, and varying political contexts.

The Role of Bureaucratic Governance

Bureaucratic governance refers to a state's ability to make and implement collectively binding decisions through an organizational structure based on standardized procedures and meritocratic recruitment. It ensures that decision-making rests in the office rather than the individual (public official) and that public employment is allocated to highly skilled professionals. This mode of governance not only lowers the risks of inefficient aid allocation and capture by narrow interests but also corresponds with openness and responsiveness, encouraging citizens to engage in accountability actions, such as monitoring activities (Hernández et al. 2019).

To assess the impact of bureaucratic governance, the next section explores whether the influence of social and political engagement on aid effectiveness is more pronounced in recipient countries with higher state capacity or whether the impact of citizen engagement persists, independent of personal networks and corruption. Specifically, the chapter examines the interaction of health aid with citizen engagement at different levels of bureaucratic governance using the State Fragility index. This index captures a country's lack of capacity to manage conflicts, design and implement public policy, and deliver essential services. If the advantageous impact of an active citizenry on health aid effectiveness is stronger in more bureaucratic states, the sign of the three-way interaction coefficient would be negative.[1] To ensure the robustness of the findings, corruption indicators from the V-Dem database, which quantify control over various forms of corruption, including public-sector corruption as well as executive, political, and regime corruption, are also used as measures of state capacity.

To measure social engagement, the analysis adheres to the methodology outlined in the preceding chapter, using the CSO Participatory Environment index to capture citizens' active participation in diverse civil-society organizations and the Social Engagement Index to assess citizens' involvement in voluntary activities and unpaid community work. The Participatory Component and the Civil Society Participation index are used to quantify elite-entrusting political engagement. Elite-challenging political engagement is measured using the Social Movement Activity index and V-Dem's Pro-Democratic and Anti-System Movement indices. These metrics not only quantify citizens' involvement in non-electoral political actions and activities of pro-democratic and anti-system opposition movements but also facilitate the distinction between protests advocating for better service delivery, the protection or expansion of democratic rights, or regime change.

Elite-Entrusting Engagement in Governance Contexts

Table 6.1 reports the estimated moderating effects of social engagement (Models 1–2) and elite-entrusting political engagement (Models 3–4) across varying contexts of bureaucratic governance. The main effect of development assistance for health (DAH) on infant mortality is significantly negative across all model specifications, which confirms the previous finding that health aid significantly reduces infant mortality at average levels of citizen involvement and bureaucratic governance. Similarly, the negative interaction between DAH and civic engagement replicates the previously identified synergistic relationship at average levels of state capacity. More importantly, the significant three-way interaction coefficients suggest significant variation in the combined effect of health aid and civic engagement between countries with low and high levels of state fragility (Models 2–4). Likewise, comparing the estimated parameters suggests similar interaction patterns for social and elite-entrusting political engagement.

The negative coefficient of Civic engagement * State fragility implies that civic engagement and state capacity are substitutes (at mean levels of health aid) regarding their effect on population health. In other words, without strong administrative capacities, increased social or political engagement is associated with lower infant mortality levels. This antagonistic interaction between civic engagement and state fragility is robust to accounting for a country's health infrastructure and the state of reproductive health care.[2] Moreover, the substitutive relationship is replicated using various measures of state capacity, including control of regime corruption, executive corruption, public-sector corruption, and political corruption (table A6.3). Given that the various corruption control measures and state fragility are inversely related, the interaction coefficients are of opposite sign, implying that civic engagement and corruption control are substitutes.

The combined effect of aid and institutions of economic governance, including control of corruption and the rule of law, has received particular attention in the aid effectiveness literature (Chauvet 2015). Thus, the results presented in table 6.1 also speak to whether state capacity directly conditions the effectiveness of development assistance. Specifically, given the main effects of health aid and state fragility, their negative interaction (DAH * State

Table 6.1. Civic Engagement, State Capacity, and Health Aid Effectiveness

	Dependent Variable: Infant Mortality Rate (Log Scale)			
	Panel 1: Social Engagement		Panel 2: Political Engagement	
	Participatory CSO Environment	Social Engagement Index	Participatory Component Index	Civil Society Participation Index
	(1)	(2)	(3)	(4)
DAH (log scale)	−0.047*** (0.015)	−0.029** (0.012)	−0.053*** (0.015)	−0.054*** (0.016)
Civic engagement	0.025** (0.010)	0.258 (0.159)	0.216*** (0.071)	0.147*** (0.045)
DAH (log scale) * Civic engagement	−0.013** (0.007)	−0.184 (0.117)	−0.134** (0.056)	−0.095*** (0.034)
State fragility	0.005 (0.005)	−0.001 (0.005)	0.008 (0.005)	0.007 (0.004)
DAH (log scale) * State fragility	−0.005*** (0.002)	−0.002* (0.001)	−0.006*** (0.002)	−0.005*** (0.002)
Civic engagement * State fragility	−0.002 (0.003)	−0.037 (0.035)	−0.010 (0.013)	−0.011 (0.010)
DAH (log scale) * Civic engagement * State fragility	−0.002 (0.001)	−0.031** (0.015)	−0.012** (0.006)	−0.012** (0.005)
IMR (lagged)	1.062*** (0.038)	1.086*** (0.034)	1.062*** (0.045)	1.063*** (0.040)
Constant	0.153 (0.308)	−0.042 (0.281)	0.143 (0.343)	0.000 (0.000)
Population (log scale)	Yes	Yes	Yes	Yes
Conflict	Yes	Yes	Yes	Yes
GDP per capita (log scale)	Yes	Yes	Yes	Yes
Period FE	Yes	Yes	Yes	Yes
Observations	479	263	479	479
Countries	124	77	124	124
Instruments	95	95	95	95
Hansen-test	0.148	0.851	0.175	0.375
AR2	0.039	0.464	0.035	0.032

Note: Table shows two-step GMM estimation with Windmeijer bias-corrected robust standard errors. Health aid (DAH) is lagged by one period. Bureaucratic governance is measured by a country's state fragility, which is inversely related to its capacity to manage conflict, make and implement public policy, and deliver essential services. Civic engagement is measured by the CSO Participatory Environment (Model 1), Social Engagement Index (Model 2), Participatory component (Model 3), and Civil Society Participation index (Model 4). DAH, bureaucratic governance, and civic engagement are mean-centered. *** p < 0.01, ** p < 0.05, * p < 0.1.

fragility) implies that health aid and administrative capacity are (imperfect) substitutes (at mean levels of civic engagement). In other words, in highly aid dependent countries, state capacity is less critical for public health, and vice versa. To put it differently, in societies with moderate civic engagement, health aid makes the largest contribution to public health in countries that have little control over corruption and are plagued by poor bureaucratic governance.

This result is consistent with the finding that corrupt recipient governments have incentives to comply with donor objectives and implement aid effectively in sectors (such as health) in which compliance is cheap to attract further external funding (Dietrich 2011). The underlying argument builds on the assumption that compliance costs are smaller in health than in other sectors because implementing health aid requires less state capacity and, at the same time, provides fewer possibilities of corruption. In sum, there is no indication that strong institutions of bureaucratic governance make health aid more effective. Instead, the evidence suggests that either state capacity or development assistance for health lowers infant mortality in recipient countries.

Yet the main question is whether the identified synergistic effect of civic engagement varies between weak and strong recipients—that is, between patronage and bureaucratic states. The significant three-way coefficients reported in table 6.1 imply substantial variation across levels of state fragility. To facilitate interpretation, figure 6.1 visualizes the estimated marginal effect of health aid across observed levels of civic engagement for recipient countries with weak, moderate, and strong administrative and organizational capacities. The short-dashed marginal effect line shows the estimated effect of health aid on infant mortality in weak patronage states as proxied by one standard deviation above the average level of state fragility. The long-dashed marginal effect line shows the same estimated effect for strong bureaucratic states as proxied by one standard deviation below the average level of state fragility. Furthermore, the solid marginal effect line indicates the interaction of health aid and civic engagement at moderate levels of state fragility.

The marginal effect plots consistently show the effect of increased health aid on infant mortality is significantly negative at higher levels of social and political engagement and is strongest in weak states. That is, the synergistic effect of civic engagement is most pronounced in states that lack the organizational and decision-making capacities to ensure adequate public-

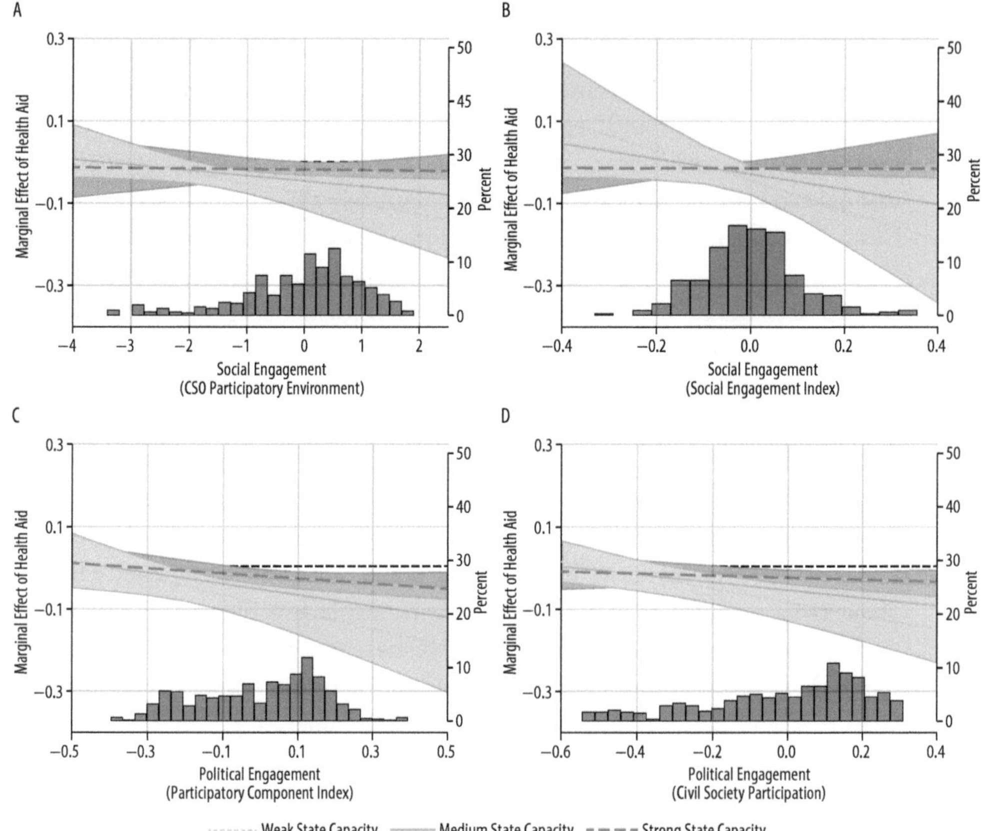

Figure 6.1. Civic Engagement, State Capacity, and the Marginal Effect of Health Aid. *Note:* Figure shows marginal effects of lagged health aid on infant mortality across the observed range of social engagement, and different state capacity levels. Plots A–D visualize the reported estimates of Model 1–4 (table 6.1). Civic engagement is measured by the CSO Participatory Environment index (A) and the Social Engagement Index (B), as well as V-Dem's Participatory Component index (C) and Civil Society Participation index (D). State capacity is measured by the State Fragility index. The solid line indicates the interaction of health aid and social engagement at mean levels of state capacity (state fragility). Weak state capacity (high state fragility) is indicated by the short-dashed line, reflecting one standard deviation below the average state capacity level. Strong state capacity (low state fragility) is indicated by the long-dashed line, reflecting one standard deviation above the average level of bureaucratic governance.

service delivery. To illustrate, in the early 2000s, a vibrant civil society in Niger converted increased international health funding into a 4 percent annual decrease in infant mortality, despite high state fragility. Conversely, in less fragile countries with an active citizenry, the marginal effect of increased health aid is lower, implying that the enhancing effects of social and political engagement are smaller or completely absent. For instance, in Costa Rica in the late 1990s, substantial increases in international health funding were associated with lower improvements in population health compared to the early 1990s, despite sustained citizen engagement and rising state capacity.

The reported differences between patronage and bureaucratic states are statistically significant, except for Model 1. But the signs of the coefficients replicate the previous finding that the enhancing effect of social engagement is strongest in weak, fragile states (figure 6.1C). Importantly, the differences are also substantially significant. In particular, in weak states with a highly involved citizenry, increases in health aid would reduce infant mortality by about twice as much as in strong states with similarly active citizens. This finding is confirmed when using alternative measures of bureaucratic governance that capture the absence of public-sector corruption as well as regime, executive, and political corruption, respectively (table A6.3). Furthermore, the results are consistent when controlling for differences in economic development, population size, involvement in conflicts, or the state of health infrastructure and reproductive health care. The findings also hold when accounting for unobserved determinants of population health using period and continent-fixed effects. This evidence consistently shows that the enhancing effect of civic engagement is strongest in countries with rampant corruption—in other words, where it is needed the most (figure A6.1).

Overall, these findings demonstrate that citizen participation can make aid work even in countries that have largely lost control of corruption. By implication, social and elite-entrusting political engagement is functionally equivalent to a bureaucratic state with the decision-making capacity and organizational competence to effectively implement development projects.

State Capacity and Elite-Challenging Engagement

The subsequent section delves into the role of elite-challenging accountability actions in the context of bureaucratic governance. To test whether the synergistic effect of citizen protest is larger in more bureaucratic, stronger states, I regress infant mortality on bureaucratic governance, health aid, and their interactions with elite-challenging political engagement. Models 1–5 focus on protests demanding regime change, while Models 6–8 look at protests advocating for the protection or strengthening of democratic freedoms. The results are documented in table 6.2.

The estimates suggest that state capacity plays an essential role in maintaining social order and security when mass movements challenge incumbents in recipient countries. Specifically, the positive sign of the three-way interaction term implies that strong bureaucratic states see the most pronounced positive effects from citizen action for accountability. In contrast, in weak and fragile states, rising citizen protest appears to diminish the effectiveness of health aid. This finding contrasts with the results from the previous analysis of social and elite-entrusting engagement.

Simultaneously, the insignificant interaction between health aid and state fragility (DAH * State fragility) suggests that even at moderate levels of social-movement activity, the capacity of a state to maintain social order helps little to strengthen aid effectiveness. This finding is consistent with the evidence presented in chapter 5, which explored the conditioning role of political institutions and formal accountability mechanisms.

Figure 6.2 shows the marginal effect of health aid on infant mortality across the observed range of elite-challenging activities in countries with weak, moderate, and strong state institutions. The figure reveals that in fragile states, the marginal effect of health aid on infant mortality is significantly negative at lower levels of elite-challenging action, but this effect diminishes as protest levels rise, as indicated by the short-dashed line. This result suggests that, in the absence of a strong state, rising social-movement activity, including pro-democratic movements and those that seek to change the entire political system, can undermine the effectiveness of health aid. The estimated effects of increased health aid in fragile states are only marginally significant, however, and thus must be interpreted with caution. In contrast, the long-dashed marginal effect line shows a negative slope, indicating that in bureaucratic states, elite-challenging activities actually boost the effectiveness of health aid. This observed effect is statistically significant across a wide range of observed social-movement activity levels and is replicated for both pro-democratic and anti-system opposition movements. Furthermore, the findings are consistent with the impact of protests advocating for better service delivery (figure A6.2, table A6.4). These results underline the role of

Table 6.2. Elite-Challenging Action, State Capacity, and Health Aid Effectiveness

	Dependent Variable: Infant Mortality Rate (Log Scale)							
	Panel 1: Anti-System Movements					Panel 2: Pro-Democratic Movements		
	(1)	(2)	(3)	(4)	(5)	(6)	(7)	(8)
DAH (log scale)	−0.034***	−0.018*	−0.027***	−0.033***	−0.022**	−0.024**	−0.028**	−0.021*
	(0.009)	(0.010)	(0.010)	(0.011)	(0.010)	(0.012)	(0.013)	(0.012)
Elite-challenging action	0.008	0.029**	0.020	−0.000	0.030**	0.025**	0.009	0.013
	(0.015)	(0.015)	(0.015)	(0.017)	(0.014)	(0.011)	(0.012)	(0.012)
DAH (log scale) * Elite-challenging action	−0.006	0.010	−0.001	0.005	0.004	0.001	0.002	−0.008
	(0.009)	(0.009)	(0.009)	(0.008)	(0.009)	(0.007)	(0.007)	(0.007)
State fragility	−0.007	−0.002	−0.004	0.004	−0.004	−0.010	0.001	−0.012*
	(0.007)	(0.005)	(0.006)	(0.006)	(0.005)	(0.006)	(0.006)	(0.007)
DAH (log scale) * State fragility	0.000	0.001	−0.000	−0.003*	0.000	−0.002	−0.003*	−0.000
	(0.001)	(0.002)	(0.001)	(0.002)	(0.001)	(0.001)	(0.002)	(0.001)
Elite-challenging action * State fragility	0.007***	0.005*	0.003	0.000	0.004**	0.004*	0.003	0.003
	(0.002)	(0.003)	(0.002)	(0.002)	(0.002)	(0.002)	(0.002)	(0.002)
DAH (log scale) * Elite-challenging action * State fragility	0.004***	0.003**	0.002**	0.002**	0.002*	0.002*	0.002**	0.003
	(0.001)	(0.001)	(0.001)	(0.001)	(0.001)	(0.001)	(0.001)	(0.002)
IMR (lagged)	1.120***	1.048***	1.075***	1.005***	1.063***	1.064***	1.017***	1.101***
	(0.043)	(0.035)	(0.043)	(0.045)	(0.037)	(0.047)	(0.059)	(0.062)
Constant	−0.341	−0.250	0.000	0.000	−0.307	0.000	−0.176	0.000
	(0.329)	(0.328)	(0.000)	(0.000)	(0.367)	(0.000)	(0.415)	(0.000)

Dependent Variable: Infant Mortality Rate (Log Scale)

	Panel 1: Anti-System Movements					Panel 2: Pro-Democratic Movements		
	(1)	(2)	(3)	(4)	(5)	(6)	(7)	(8)
Period FE	Yes	Yes	Yes	Yes	Yes	Yes	Yes	Yes
Conflict	Yes	Yes	Yes	Yes	Yes	Yes	Yes	Yes
GDP per capita (log scale)	Yes	Yes	Yes	Yes	Yes	Yes	Yes	Yes
Population (log scale)	Yes	Yes	Yes	Yes	Yes	Yes	Yes	Yes
Female education		Yes	Yes	Yes	Yes	Yes	Yes	Yes
Physicians (log scale)		Yes			Yes			Yes
Fertility rate (log scale)			Yes		Yes	Yes		Yes
HIV prevalence (log scale)				Yes			Yes	
Observations	479	341	389	322	341	301	245	266
Countries	124	101	101	82	101	81	65	80
Instruments	87	105	105	105	114	105	105	114
Hansen-test	0.028	0.362	0.310	0.920	0.676	0.945	0.999	0.969
AR2	0.202	0.112	0.249	0.052	0.126	0.545	0.867	0.917

Note: Table shows two-step GMM estimation with Windmeijer bias-corrected robust standard errors. Elite-challenging action is measured by Anti-System Movements (Models 1–5) and Pro-Democratic Movements (Models 6–8). Bureaucratic governance is measured by the state fragility index. Health aid (DAH) is lagged by one period. DAH, bureaucratic governance, and elite-challenging action are mean-centered. *** $p<0.01$, ** $p<0.05$, * $p<0.1$.

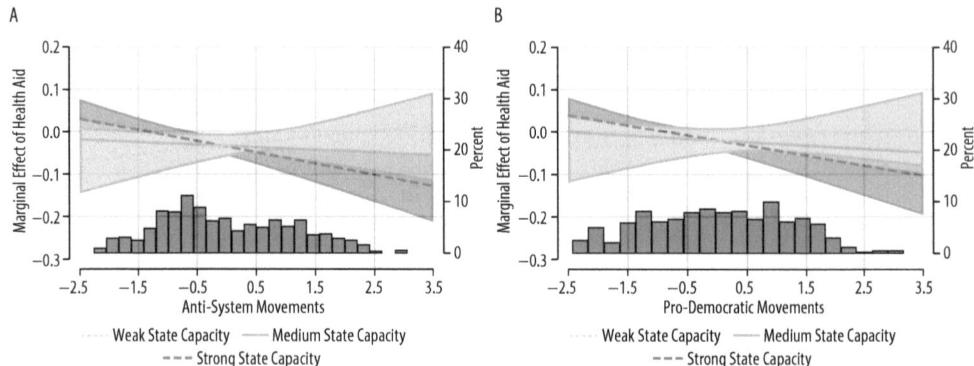

Figure 6.2. Elite-Challenging Action, State Capacity, and the Marginal Effect of Health Aid. *Note:* Figure shows the average marginal effect of increased health aid across different levels of elite-challenging action and bureaucratic governance. The plot visualizes the reported estimates of Model 1 and 8 (table 6.2). Elite-challenging action is measured by the (A) Anti-System Movements and (B) Pro-Democratic Movements indices. Bureaucratic governance is measured by a country's level of state fragility. Health aid (DAH) is lagged by one period. DAH, bureaucratic governance, and elite-challenging action are mean-centered.

state capacity in preventing citizen demand through mass movements from undermining security and destabilizing central authority. Notably, these findings hold after controlling for additional socioeconomic and sociopolitical determinants, including the state of reproductive health care, women's education, HIV prevalence, and the quality of health infrastructure.

To illustrate, during the late 1990s and early 2000s, Mauritius, being one of the least-fragile states in sub-Saharan Africa with high administrative and organizational capacities, ensured the government maintained social order and responded to demands from democratic mass movements, converting substantial amounts of health aid per capita into an over 3 percent annual reduction in infant mortality. Conversely, in the early 1990s, the Democratic Republic of the Congo experienced a starkly different reality. Hindered by a lack of state capacity and widespread corruption, the government failed to respond to increased citizen demands and effectively use international health funding to improve population health. In sum, higher state capacity ensures that citizens' political engagement in elite-challenging activities enhances aid effectiveness without jeopardizing regime stability.

Moreover, it equips authorities with the required organizational and decision-making capacities to address increased citizen demands.

The study's results complement research on social movements in African countries. For instance, Harris and Hern (2018) find that in regimes where formal avenues of political engagement are insufficient for communicating preferences to the government, citizens who expect governments to be responsive are more likely to protest and demand better service delivery. The present findings suggest that states' capacity to maintain social order and address citizen demands ensures that elite-challenging political engagement enhances aid effectiveness and prevents the destabilization of political authority.

In conclusion, the influence of social engagement on aid effectiveness varies markedly between weak patronage and strong bureaucratic states. In weaker states plagued by rampant corruption, social engagement can make health aid more effective despite the absence of strong state institutions. In contrast, this enhancing effect is less pronounced in bureaucratic states. These findings challenge Hypothesis 2a, formulated in chapter 2, which posited that the enhancing effect of social engagement is stronger in countries with greater state capacity. Rather, the evidence suggests that social engagement has the largest payoff in recipient countries with dysfunctional state institutions. Consequently, the weaker a state's decision-making and organizational capacity, the more important social engagement becomes in bolstering health aid effectiveness.

These results resonate with evidence from comparative research on state capacity in developing countries and areas of limited statehood, demonstrating that the provision of public goods and services does not necessarily depend on functioning state institutions (Börzel and Risse 2016, 149). The findings are also supported by case-study evidence showing that traditional, self-governing organizations can maintain political order and deliver public goods, even in fragile and conflict-ridden contexts like Afghanistan (Murtazashvili 2016).

Regarding the enhancing effects of political engagement, the role of the governance context varies between elite-entrusting and elite-challenging modes of citizen participation. On the one hand, evidence suggests that a politically engaged citizenry, capable of converting activism into political power, can enhance the effectiveness of health aid even when strong state institutions are absent, contradicting Hypothesis 2b. On the other hand, there is striking evidence that increased elite-challenging political activities only enhance health aid effectiveness as long as states are able to maintain social order and respond to citizen demands. In fragile states, where political authorities are persistently challenged and unable to control political violence and ensure security, increased social-movement activity thus undermines health aid effectiveness. This finding supports Hypothesis 2c, which posits that bureaucratic governance strengthens the enhancing effect of elite-challenging political engagement on making aid work.

The Role of Liberal Democracy

Democratic institutions inherently shape citizen demand for accountability and government responsiveness by creating specific incentives. Freedom of expression and association, for example, mitigate the individual costs of engaging in elite-challenging actions, while media independence allows civil society to articulate demands and communicate outcomes of investigations by oversight institutions. Furthermore, free and fair elections allow citizens to penalize poor health-service delivery and indirectly exercise accountability over implementing agencies. The effectiveness of citizen action for accountability ultimately depends, however, on a judiciary and legislature that operate independently and have the authority to prosecute illegal behavior—because "voice needs teeth to have a bite" (Fox 2015, 357). Therefore, formally institutionalized oversight mechanisms, guaranteeing judicial and legislative independence, are expected to strengthen the enhancing effect of citizen demand for accountability on making aid more effective. Thus, health aid is hypothesized to improve population health, especially in recipient countries with an active citizenry and strong democratic oversight institutions.

The subsequent section examines whether the quality of democracy influences the synergistic interaction between civic engagement and health aid, as previously identified. Various composite indices of democracy, along with specific indicators of accountability and executive oversight, are employed to assess the role of democratic institutions. The composite democracy indices used include the Freedom House (FH) index and the Coalition to Selectorate Size (CSS) ratio. The FH index captures the presence of political rights and civil liberties, while the CSS ratio directly measures politicians' incentives to provide public goods based on the extent of open and competitive executive recruitment, party competition, and the legislature's independence. Additionally, the binary Democracy vs. Dictatorship indicator, introduced by Cheibub, Gandhi, and Vreeland (2010), captures electoral accountability based on free and fair elections and multiparty competition. A selection of V-Dem indicators measures the extent of oversight on the executive by the legislature, governmental oversight agencies (from an ombudsperson or general prosecutor), and non-state institutions.

Elite-Entrusting Engagement in Democratic Contexts

Table 6.3 details the varying effects of social and elite-entrusting political engagement across different levels of liberal democracy. Consistent with previous findings, the main effect of health aid is significantly negative throughout all model specifications. The reported negative interaction term of DAH and civic engagement replicates the synergistic effects of social and political involvement identified earlier, although the coefficient is consistently insignificant. This suggests that in moderately democratic recipient countries, civic engagement does not significantly enhance the effectiveness of health aid.

Instead, there is indication that the impact of civic engagement is more pronounced in authoritarian countries. Specifically, the patterns observed across different model specifications and democracy measures suggest the enhancing effects of social and political engagement are somewhat stronger in less democratic states. But only the interaction between political engagement and democratic oversight in Models 8 and 10 achieves conventional levels of statistical significance. Thus, these results imply that democratic oversight mechanisms do not generally strengthen the impact of social and elite-entrusting political engagement on aid effectiveness.[3] Instead, evidence suggests that civic engagement can enhance the effectiveness of health aid, even in less democratic settings, as illustrated by figure 6.3.

Figure 6.3 shows the marginal effects of lagged health aid on infant mortality across the observed range of political engagement and democratic oversight. Notably, even in the least democratic country, as illustrated by the short-dashed sloping line, higher civic engagement is correlated with increased aid effectiveness. The marginal effect plots reveal that a politically active citizenry can substantially strengthen the effectiveness of health aid, even when (A) formal mechanisms of accountability and democratic oversight are weak, or (B) the legislature is not independent, and party competition is limited.

Table 6.3. Civic Engagement, Liberal Democracy, and Health Aid Effectiveness

	Dependent Variable: Infant Mortality Rate (Log Scale)									
	Panel 1: Social Engagement					Panel 2: Political Engagement				
	Legislative Constraints	Executive Oversight	Gov. Accountability	Freedom House	CSS Ratio	Legislative Constraints	Executive Oversight	Gov. Accountability	Freedom House	CSS Ratio
	(1)	(2)	(3)	(4)	(5)	(6)	(7)	(8)	(9)	(10)
DAH (log scale)	−0.035***	−0.026**	−0.036***	−0.029***	−0.027**	−0.029**	−0.021	−0.044***	−0.044***	−0.038***
	(0.013)	(0.013)	(0.010)	(0.011)	(0.011)	(0.011)	(0.013)	(0.010)	(0.014)	(0.014)
Civic engagement	0.051***	0.079***	0.073***	0.055**	0.037**	0.133	0.150	0.232**	0.243**	0.265***
	(0.019)	(0.023)	(0.025)	(0.022)	(0.018)	(0.107)	(0.131)	(0.107)	(0.116)	(0.103)
DAH (log scale) * Civic engagement	−0.007	0.003	−0.004	−0.002	−0.008	−0.073*	−0.054	−0.095	−0.079	−0.050
	(0.010)	(0.008)	(0.010)	(0.011)	(0.009)	(0.039)	(0.049)	(0.099)	(0.124)	(0.073)
Liberal democracy	0.024	−0.002	−0.006	0.066	−0.097	0.043	−0.011	−0.001	0.024	−0.163**
	(0.074)	(0.015)	(0.037)	(0.088)	(0.065)	(0.064)	(0.017)	(0.031)	(0.073)	(0.077)
DAH (log scale) * Liberal democracy	0.009	−0.009	0.011	0.006	−0.001	0.030	−0.000	0.019	0.057	−0.024
	(0.041)	(0.010)	(0.012)	(0.034)	(0.043)	(0.024)	(0.008)	(0.020)	(0.073)	(0.051)
Civic engagement * Liberal democracy	0.097***	0.029***	0.028***	0.095**	0.064	−0.063	−0.030	0.018	0.156	0.563
	(0.031)	(0.008)	(0.010)	(0.040)	(0.061)	(0.217)	(0.066)	(0.067)	(0.208)	(0.529)
DAH (log scale) * Civic engagement * Liberal democracy	0.021	0.004	0.008	0.021	0.007	0.111	0.023	0.104***	0.269	0.382*
	(0.032)	(0.007)	(0.006)	(0.022)	(0.032)	(0.135)	(0.044)	(0.033)	(0.172)	(0.201)
IMR (lagged)	1.074***	1.017***	1.049***	1.051***	1.055***	1.126***	1.091***	1.110***	1.104***	1.082***
	(0.043)	(0.041)	(0.045)	(0.047)	(0.038)	(0.039)	(0.035)	(0.037)	(0.030)	(0.036)

| Dependent Variable: Infant Mortality Rate (Log Scale) | | | | | | | | | |
Panel 1: Social Engagement					Panel 2: Political Engagement				
Legislative Constraints	Executive Oversight	Gov. Accountability	Freedom House	CSS Ratio	Legislative Constraints	Executive Oversight	Gov. Accountability	Freedom House	CSS Ratio
(1)	(2)	(3)	(4)	(5)	(6)	(7)	(8)	(9)	(10)

	(1)	(2)	(3)	(4)	(5)	(6)	(7)	(8)	(9)	(10)
Constant	0.104 (0.340)	0.000 (0.000)	0.000 (0.000)	0.000 (0.000)	0.000 (0.000)	0.000 (0.000)	0.000 (0.000)	−0.253 (0.325)	0.000 (0.000)	0.000 (0.000)
Period FE	Yes	Yes	Yes	Yes	Yes	Yes	Yes	Yes	Yes	Yes
Conflict	Yes	Yes	Yes	Yes	Yes	Yes	Yes	Yes	Yes	Yes
Population (log scale)	Yes	Yes	Yes	Yes	Yes	Yes	Yes	Yes	Yes	Yes
GDP (log scale)	Yes	Yes	Yes	Yes	Yes	Yes	Yes	Yes	Yes	Yes
Public-sector corruption	Yes	Yes	Yes	Yes	Yes	Yes	Yes	Yes	Yes	Yes
Observations	481	481	484	484	483	481	481	484	484	483
Countries	125	125	125	125	125	125	125	125	125	125
Instruments	95	95	95	95	95	95	95	95	95	95
Hansen-test	0.080	0.117	0.094	0.065	0.034	0.046	0.100	0.136	0.240	0.072
AR2	0.410	0.528	0.279	0.257	0.255	0.184	0.240	0.144	0.096	0.179

Note: Table shows two-step GMM estimation with Windmeijer bias-corrected robust standard errors. Social engagement is measured by the CSO Participatory Environment index. Political engagement is measured by the Civil Society Participation index. Liberal democracy is measured by the Legislative Constraints index (M1 and M6), Executive Oversight index (M2 and M7), Government Accountability index (M3 and M8), Freedom House index (M4 and M9), and the CSS Ratio (M5 and M10). Health aid (DAH) is lagged by one period. DAH, civic engagement, and liberal democracy are mean-centered. *** p<0.01, ** p<0.05, * p<0.1.

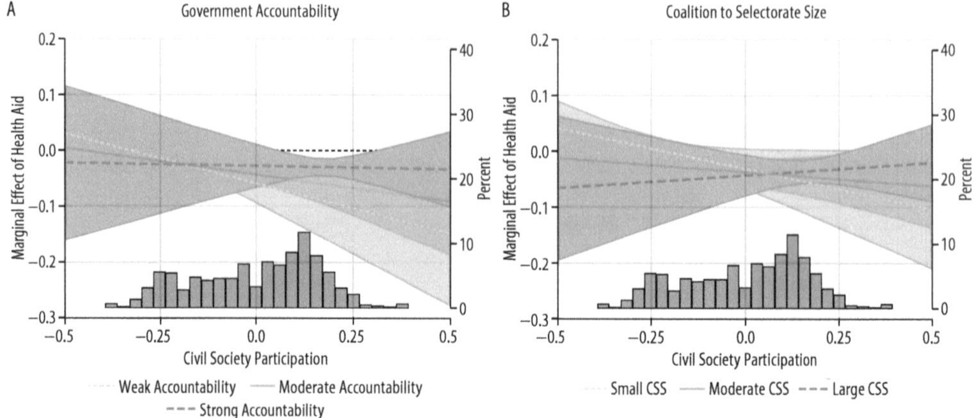

Figure 6.3. **Political Engagement, Democracy, and the Marginal Effect of Health Aid.** *Note:* Figure shows marginal effects of lagged health aid on infant mortality across the observed range of political engagement and for different levels of democratic oversight. Plots A and B visualize the estimates of Models 8 and 10 reported in table 6.3. Political engagement is measured by the Civil Society Participation index. Democratic oversight institutions are measured using the Government Accountability index (A) and the Coalition to Selectorate Size (CSS) ratio (B). The solid line indicates the interaction of health aid and political engagement at mean levels of democracy. Regimes with weak democratic oversight are indicated by the short-dashed line (reflecting one standard deviation below the mean). Regimes with strong democratic oversight are indicated by the long-dashed line (reflecting one standard deviation above the mean). Health aid (DAH) is lagged by one period.

To illustrate, in the early 2000s, a politically active citizenry enabled Vietnam to convert increased international health funding into an annual decline in infant mortality of about 3 percent despite the absence of robust formal accountability mechanisms. Similarly, in the late 2000s, Uganda, with its politically engaged citizenry, translated rising health aid into a 6 percent annual decrease in infant mortality despite the lack of an independent legislature and restricted party competition. In contrast, in countries with strong democratic oversight institutions like South Africa in the early 2000s, increases in health funding did not result in improved population health despite a vibrant civil society.

Consequently, even if democratic institutions are absent, increased social and elite-entrusting political engagement can make aid work better.

Conversely, in recipient countries with strong democratic oversight institutions, increased citizen involvement does not significantly impact the effectiveness of health aid, as depicted by the nearly horizontal long-dashed sloping line in figure 6.3.

The evidence presented in this section suggests the impact of social and elite-entrusting political engagement varies little between autocracies and democracies. Together with the findings of chapter 5, these results imply that formally institutionalized democratic oversight mechanisms do not necessarily strengthen the impact of civic engagement on aid effectiveness.[4] Hence, there is no indication that democracy generally strengthens the impact of civic engagement on aid effectiveness. On the contrary, increased elite-entrusting political engagement appears to improve the effectiveness of health aid, even in the absence of democratic institutions, disproving Hypotheses 3a and 3b.

Democratic Institutions and Elite-Challenging Engagement

How does elite-challenging political engagement influence aid effectiveness in the context of democratic governance? Where democratic institutions ensure formal oversight and create incentives for citizen demand and government responsiveness, they are likely to strengthen the enhancing impact of citizen protest on the effectiveness of health aid. For instance, between 2005 and 2013, Ghana—one of the most democratic recipient countries in sub-Saharan Africa—saw over 3 percent annual reduction in infant mortality amid significant health funding and strong pro-democratic mass movements. Conversely, where democratic institutions are absent, like in Zimbabwe in the early 2000s, political engagement is likely to render health aid less effective, with political leaders misusing foreign aid to suppress movements that pose a threat to regime stability. To explore whether the synergistic impact of citizen protest is more pronounced in democracies, infant mortality is regressed on different measures of democratic oversight, health aid, and their interactions with political engagement, as detailed in table 6.4.

The estimates highlight the pivotal role of democratic institutions in leveraging the impact of political engagement on aid effectiveness. Notably, the coefficient of the three-way interaction indicates significant differences between democratic and authoritarian regimes. The data further suggests a synergistic relationship between citizen participation in elite-challenging

Table 6.4. Elite-Challenging Action, Liberal Democracy, and Health Aid Effectiveness

	Dependent Variable: Infant Mortality Rate (Log Scale)									
	Freedom House		CSS Ratio		Democracy vs. Dictatorship		Executive Oversight		Horizontal Accountability	
	(1)	(2)	(3)	(4)	(5)	(6)	(7)	(8)	(9)	(10)
DAH (log scale)	−0.014	−0.014*	−0.011	−0.009	0.013	0.009	0.000	−0.002	−0.009	−0.007
	(0.011)	(0.008)	(0.009)	(0.008)	(0.015)	(0.011)	(0.012)	(0.010)	(0.011)	(0.010)
Elite-challenging action	0.002	−0.002	0.025**	0.022*	0.029	0.031*	0.025**	0.021	0.029**	0.029*
	(0.013)	(0.012)	(0.012)	(0.012)	(0.020)	(0.018)	(0.013)	(0.014)	(0.013)	(0.015)
DAH (log scale) * Elite-challenging action	−0.010	−0.010	−0.004	−0.006	0.018**	0.012	0.001	−0.002	−0.006	−0.006
	(0.009)	(0.008)	(0.006)	(0.006)	(0.008)	(0.008)	(0.009)	(0.008)	(0.008)	(0.008)
Liberal democracy	0.104*	0.122**	−0.110	−0.096	−0.016	−0.014	−0.002	0.009	0.001	0.011
	(0.060)	(0.057)	(0.070)	(0.087)	(0.029)	(0.027)	(0.019)	(0.019)	(0.031)	(0.027)
DAH (log scale) * Liberal democracy	−0.045*	−0.044*	−0.084***	−0.078***	−0.034*	−0.033**	−0.025**	−0.021***	−0.028**	−0.023**
	(0.027)	(0.025)	(0.027)	(0.024)	(0.019)	(0.016)	(0.010)	(0.008)	(0.011)	(0.010)
Elite-challenging action * Liberal democracy	−0.010	−0.025	−0.075*	−0.062	−0.023	−0.027	0.008	0.007	0.000	0.002
	(0.028)	(0.030)	(0.039)	(0.038)	(0.023)	(0.026)	(0.008)	(0.007)	(0.015)	(0.012)
DAH (log scale) * Elite-challenging action * Liberal democracy	−0.072**	−0.063**	−0.052**	−0.052**	−0.048***	−0.041***	−0.017**	−0.014**	−0.025***	−0.021***
	(0.029)	(0.029)	(0.023)	(0.026)	(0.014)	(0.016)	(0.007)	(0.007)	(0.008)	(0.008)
IMR (lagged)	1.097***	1.074***	1.118***	1.097***	1.110***	1.110***	1.089***	1.086***	1.103***	1.086***
	(0.045)	(0.042)	(0.042)	(0.042)	(0.047)	(0.057)	(0.050)	(0.057)	(0.055)	(0.047)
Constant	−0.701*	0.000	−0.791***	−0.708***	−0.748***	0.000	0.000	−0.775**	−0.659	−0.666**
	(0.374)	(0.000)	(0.290)	(0.261)	(0.264)	(0.000)	(0.000)	(0.385)	(0.403)	(0.302)

	Dependent Variable: Infant Mortality Rate (Log Scale)									
	Freedom House		CSS Ratio		Democracy vs. Dictatorship		Executive Oversight		Horizontal Accountability	
	(1)	(2)	(3)	(4)	(5)	(6)	(7)	(8)	(9)	(10)
Period FE	Yes	Yes	Yes	Yes	Yes	Yes	Yes	Yes	Yes	Yes
Conflict	Yes	Yes	Yes	Yes	Yes	Yes	Yes	Yes	Yes	Yes
GDP per capita (log scale)	Yes	Yes	Yes	Yes	Yes	Yes	Yes	Yes	Yes	Yes
Population (log scale)	Yes	Yes	Yes	Yes	Yes	Yes	Yes	Yes	Yes	Yes
Public-sector corruption control	Yes	Yes	Yes	Yes	Yes	Yes	Yes	Yes	Yes	Yes
Physicians (log scale)	Yes	Yes	Yes	Yes	Yes	Yes	Yes	Yes	Yes	Yes
Fertility rate (log scale)		Yes		Yes		Yes		Yes		Yes
Observations	333	333	332	332	333	333	332	332	333	333
Countries	99	99	99	99	99	99	99	99	99	99
Instruments	105	105	105	114	105	114	105	114	105	114
Hansen-test	0.376	0.569	0.367	0.703	0.405	0.750	0.451	0.732	0.337	0.668
AR2	0.980	0.805	0.806	0.929	0.948	0.876	0.768	0.933	0.709	0.794

Note: Table shows two-step GMM estimation with Windmeijer bias-corrected robust standard errors. Elite-challenging action is measured by the Pro-Democratic Movements index. Liberal democracy is measured by the Freedom House index (Models 1 and 2), the CSS ratio (Models 3 and 4), and the Democracy vs. Dictatorship (Models 5 and 6), Executive Oversight (Models 7 and 8), and Horizontal Accountability (Models 9–10) indices. Health aid (DAH) is lagged by one period. DAH, elite-challenging action, and liberal democracy are mean-centered. *** $p < 0.01$, ** $p < 0.05$, * $p < 0.1$.

activities and democratic institutions. Together, these results imply that democracy strengthens the enhancing impact of elite-challenging engagement on the effectiveness of health aid, confirming Hypothesis 3c.

Notably, this finding is consistent across diverse democracy measures, with the Freedom House index of political rights and civil liberties bringing about the largest impact of political engagement on aid effectiveness (Models 1–2).[5] Moreover, democratic institutions that ensure legislative independence, open and competitive executive recruitment, and party competition (Models 3–6), as well as specific institutionalized horizontal oversight mechanisms (Models 7–10), also strengthen the synergistic effect of elite-challenging mass movements on making aid work better.

To facilitate interpretation, figure 6.4 displays the estimated marginal effect of health aid across observed levels of elite-challenging action for recipient countries with weak, moderate, and strong democratic institutions.[6] All plots consistently show that, if democratic institutions are in place, the effect of health aid on infant mortality is significantly negative and grows as levels of elite-challenging action rise, as evidenced by the negatively sloped long-dashed marginal effect lines. Increased elite-challenging action enhances the effectiveness of health aid in states where (A) political rights and civil liberties are guaranteed, (B) executive actions are subject to oversight, (C) elections are held, and parties compete for political influence, and (D) the government is held accountable by different oversight bodies. Importantly, this finding holds after accounting for states' capacity to maintain social order and security.

In democracies, the impact of elite-challenging engagement is substantially higher than in their authoritarian counterparts. Specifically, in an otherwise average recipient country with high levels of elite-challenging mass movements, doubling health aid would lower infant mortality by about 3 percent (see table 5.3). For a democratic recipient with an equally active citizenry (and all else being constant), the same increase in development assistance would reduce the mortality rate by about 5 to 6 percent. Conversely, in non-democracies, rising levels of elite-challenging action render aid ineffective. Thus, given similar levels of elite-challenging engagement, the effectiveness of health aid in authoritarian countries is lower than in their democratic counterparts. By implication, the lack of democratic institutions undermines the enhancing impact of elite-challenging actions that help to make health aid work better. This finding is consistent

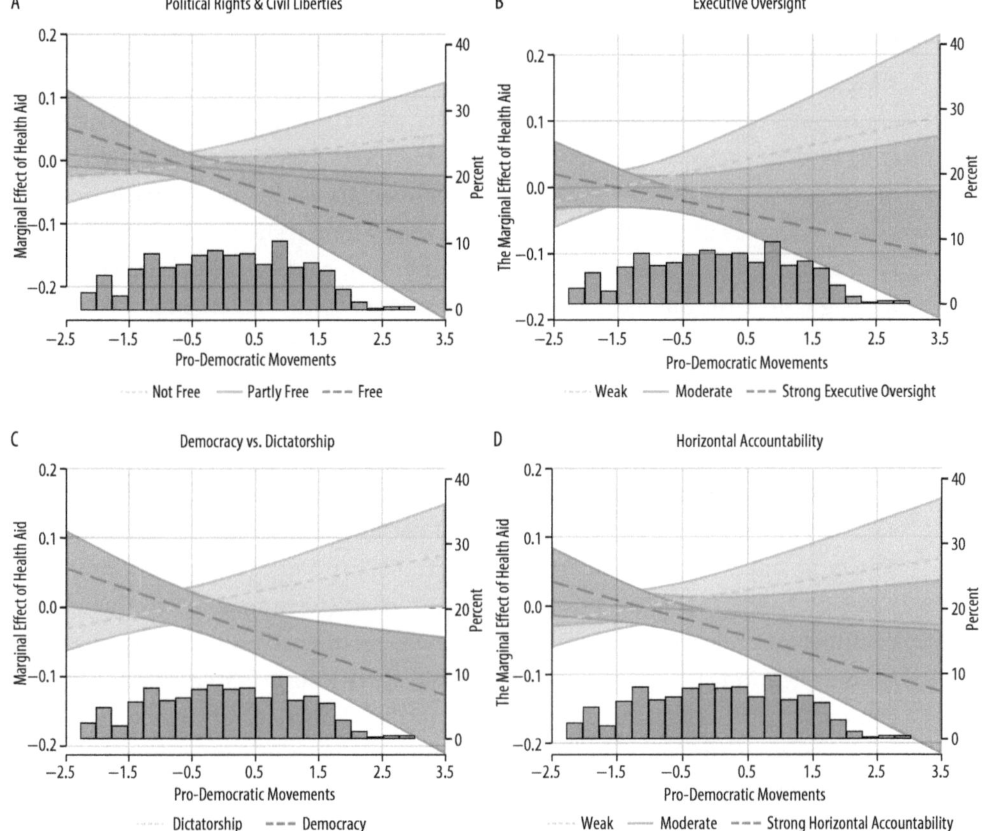

Figure 6.4. Elite-Challenging Action, Democracy, and the Marginal Effect of Health Aid. *Note:* Figure shows marginal effects of lagged health aid on infant mortality across the observed range of elite-challenging action and for different levels of democracy. Plots A–D visualize the reported estimates of Models 1, 5, 7, and 9 reported in table 6.4. Elite-challenging action is measured by the Pro-Democratic Movements index. Democracy is measured by the Freedom House index (A), Executive Oversight index (B), Democracy vs. Dictatorship index (C), and the Horizontal Accountability index (D). The solid line indicates the interaction of health aid and political engagement at mean levels of democracy. Regimes classified as "not free" or dictatorships and countries with weak executive oversight or weak horizontal accountability are indicated by the short-dashed line (reflecting one standard deviation below the mean). Democracies, regimes classified as "free," and countries with strong executive oversight or strong horizontal accountability are indicated by the long-dashed line (reflecting one standard deviation above the mean). Health aid (DAH) is lagged by one period.

with the claim that authoritarian leaders facing mass movements are likely to divert aid away from its intended purposes to lower the threat of a regime change.

Importantly, these results are consistent with the impact of less ideologically driven movements, including elite-challenging actions advocating for better service delivery or regime change. Across various democracy measures and subsamples of aid recipients, various robustness tests, detailed in table A6.6 and table A6.7 and illustrated in figure A6.3, confirm that democratic oversight institutions strengthen the impact of elite-challenging engagement on the effectiveness of health aid. In summary, elite-challenging actions exert the largest impact on health aid effectiveness in democratic countries, while authoritarian institutions subvert the enhancing effects of citizen-led accountability action, undermining health aid effectiveness.

This subchapter examined whether formal institutions of liberal democracy strengthen the enhancing effects of social and political engagement. The reported evidence indicates no discernible difference between democracies and autocracies concerning the extent to which elite-entrusting forms of citizen participation enhance the effectiveness of health aid. Hence, there is no indication the presence of democratic institutions fosters the synergistic effect of noncontentious forms of social and political engagement. Instead, even in the least democratic environment, social and particularly elite-entrusting political engagement can make aid work better. Based on these results, Hypotheses 3a and 3b are rejected.

Differences emerge between autocracies and democracies concerning elite-challenging forms of political engagement, however. In particular, the identified synergistic effect of elite-challenging actions is strongest in states where democratic rights are guaranteed. This finding supports Hypothesis 3c, positing that democratic oversight institutions strengthen the impact of elite-challenging engagement on aid effectiveness. Conversely, in autocracies, rising levels of contentious political behavior are associated with increased ineffectiveness of development assistance. This finding is consistent with recent evidence from research on comparative authoritarianism (Bueno de Mesquita and Smith 2009; 2010) and is also corroborated by qualitative research on the adverse outcomes of citizen action for accountability, such as violent state responses or the denial of state services and resources (Gaventa and Barrett 2012; Evans and Heller 2015).

The Role of Decentralization

Decentralization reduces the distance between governments and citizens, enabling service users to articulate their needs and preferences to local representatives and have a real say in planning and implementing local development projects. Additionally, decentralization creates incentives for local officials to respond to those they are supposed to serve and by whom they are elected, shifting their focus away from central government priorities. Consequently, in decentralized countries, local officials are not only better informed about the demands of a heterogeneous population but also more subject to public scrutiny than national governments. Given these incentives, decentralization is expected to strengthen the enhancing impact of an active citizenry. By implication, health aid is hypothesized to have a more positive effect on population health in decentralized recipient countries with a vibrant voluntary sector. The subsequent section examines the impact of social and political engagement on the effectiveness of health aid in decentralized contexts.

While decentralization is a multidimensional process of transferring power, responsibilities, and resources from central to local authorities, this study focuses on administrative and political decentralization because of a lack of data on fiscal decentralization. The transfer of decision-making authority and responsibility to the local level is measured by the extent of subnational governments' authority over taxing, spending, and regulation. Similarly, the transfer of legislative and executive power to subnational units is captured by a set of V-Dem indicators, measuring whether regional and local governments exist, whether they are elected, and the extent to which they can operate without interference from unelected local bodies.

Elite-Entrusting Engagement in Decentralized Contexts

Table 6.5 reports the estimated moderating effects of social engagement (panel 1) and elite-entrusting political engagement (panel 2) in the context of political and administrative decentralization. Supporting previous findings, the effect of health aid and its interaction with civic engagement is significantly negative across all model specifications, implying that increased citizen involvement in moderately decentralized countries makes health aid more effective. At the same time, the coefficients of decentralization and its interaction with health aid imply that the transfer of power and authority

Table 6.5. Civic Engagement, Decentralization, and Health Aid Effectiveness

	Dependent Variable: Infant Mortality Rate (Log Scale)						
	Panel 1: Social Engagement			Panel 2: Political Engagement			
	Power of Local Governments	Locally Elected Executive/ Legislature	Local Government Index	Power of Local Governments	Power of Regional Governments	Locally Elected Executive/ Legislature	Subnational Authority over Taxing
	(1)	(2)	(3)	(4)	(5)	(6)	(7)
DAH (log scale)	−0.040***	−0.047**	−0.035***	−0.042***	−0.073***	−0.039**	−0.023**
	(0.009)	(0.021)	(0.009)	(0.010)	(0.012)	(0.018)	(0.011)
Civic engagement	0.010	0.023	0.024	0.163*	0.204*	0.241**	0.148
	(0.013)	(0.020)	(0.019)	(0.095)	(0.109)	(0.104)	(0.117)
DAH (log scale) * Civic engagement	−0.019***	−0.025**	−0.008	−0.087**	−0.135**	−0.106**	−0.051*
	(0.006)	(0.010)	(0.007)	(0.044)	(0.068)	(0.054)	(0.030)
Decentralization	0.017	−0.073**	−0.006	0.013	0.013	−0.084**	0.060
	(0.012)	(0.032)	(0.045)	(0.014)	(0.016)	(0.036)	(0.038)
DAH (log scale) * Decentralization	0.018**	0.022	0.011	0.013	0.024**	0.014	−0.000
	(0.008)	(0.024)	(0.026)	(0.008)	(0.012)	(0.019)	(0.015)
Civic engagement * Decentralization	−0.005	0.043	0.026	−0.006	−0.017	0.281**	0.081
	(0.007)	(0.029)	(0.036)	(0.042)	(0.039)	(0.115)	(0.210)
DAH (log scale) * Civic engagement * Decentralization	0.009*	0.022*	0.039*	0.037*	0.091***	0.135**	0.216***
	(0.005)	(0.012)	(0.024)	(0.019)	(0.029)	(0.068)	(0.076)
IMR (lagged)	1.027***	1.060***	1.051***	1.061***	1.083***	1.034***	1.023***
	(0.027)	(0.043)	(0.044)	(0.040)	(0.043)	(0.054)	(0.040)
Constant	0.029	0.000	0.000	0.000	0.282	0.239	0.283
	(0.237)	(0.000)	(0.000)	(0.000)	(0.331)	(0.443)	(0.363)

	Dependent Variable: Infant Mortality Rate (Log Scale)						
	Panel 1: Social Engagement			Panel 2: Political Engagement			
	Power of Local Governments	Locally Elected Executive/ Legislature	Local Government Index	Power of Local Governments	Power of Regional Governments	Locally Elected Executive/ Legislature	Subnational Authority over Taxing
	(1)	(2)	(3)	(4)	(5)	(6)	(7)
Period FE	Yes	Yes	Yes	Yes	Yes	Yes	Yes
Conflict	Yes	Yes	Yes	Yes	Yes	Yes	Yes
Population (log scale)	Yes	Yes	Yes	Yes	Yes	Yes	Yes
GDP (log scale)	Yes	Yes	Yes	Yes	Yes	Yes	Yes
Public-sector corruption	Yes	Yes	Yes	Yes	Yes	Yes	Yes
Fertility rate (log scale)	Yes	Yes					
Physicians (log scale)			Yes				
Observations	473	374	421	473	409	374	179
Countries	124	99	123	124	107	99	47
Instruments	104	104	104	95	95	95	92
Hansen-test	0.256	0.188	0.120	0.105	0.312	0.074	0.999
AR2	0.197	0.306	0.140	0.383	0.184	0.428	0.269

Note: Table shows two-step GMM estimation with Windmeijer bias-corrected robust standard errors. Social engagement is measured by the CSO Participatory Environment index (panel 1). Political engagement is measured by the Civil Society Participation index (panel 2). Decentralization captures local or regional governments' relative power (M1, M4, M5), whether local offices of the executive or legislature are locally elected (M2 and M6) or whether subnational governments have authority over taxing, spending, and legislation (M7). Health aid (DAH) is lagged by one period. DAH, civic engagement, and decentralization are mean-centered. *** $p < 0.01$, ** $p < 0.05$, * $p < 0.1$.

to the local level does not directly lower infant mortality, nor does it make aid more effective. The three-way interaction term is statistically significant across all model specifications, however, suggesting the combined effect of both social and political engagement with health aid varies significantly across observed levels of decentralization. This result is replicated across different measures of political and administrative decentralization and holds after accounting for differences in economic development, population size, conflict involvement, public-sector corruption, health infrastructure, reproductive health care, and period effects. The positive sign of the interaction coefficient further implies that social and elite-entrusting political engagement makes health aid more effective, particularly in weakly decentralized countries. That is, the transfer of power and responsibilities to the local level seems to weaken the enhancing effects of civic engagement.

To further explore the reported estimates, figure 6.5 displays the marginal effects of health aid across observed levels of social engagement and political decentralization. The varying levels of political decentralization reflect (A) differences in local offices' relative power and (B) differences between offices that are locally elected and those that are not. The figure shows that, in countries with an active citizenry, the negative effect of health aid on infant mortality is strongest if authority is firmly centralized. In particular, the large negative slope of the short-dashed marginal effect line (A) indicates that social engagement makes health aid most effective in weakly decentralized recipient countries (one standard deviation below the mean) where local officeholders are less autonomous. Conversely, the flat long-dashed marginal effect line implies that, in strongly decentralized recipient countries (one standard deviation above the mean level) that have transferred authority and power to locally elected offices, the enhancing effect of social engagement is smaller than in countries with less autonomous subnational governments. Notably, in centralized states with a highly active citizenry, increases in health aid would reduce infant mortality by about three times as much as in decentralized states with equally active citizens.

Similarly, in recipient countries with locally elected executives or legislatures, social engagement fails to significantly enhance the effectiveness of health aid, as depicted by the nearly horizontal long-dashed marginal effect line in plot B. To illustrate, the Republic of the Congo's decentralization efforts in the first half of the 1990s coincided with annual declines in

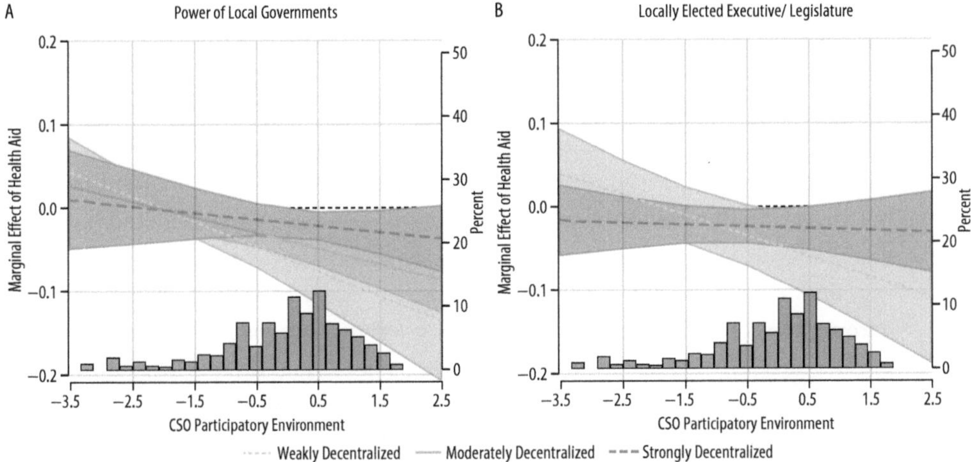

Figure 6.5. Social Engagement, Decentralization, and the Marginal Effect of Health Aid. *Note:* Figure shows average marginal effects of lagged health aid on infant mortality across the observed range of social engagement and decentralization. Plots A and B visualize the estimates of Models 1 and 2 reported in table 6.5. Social engagement is measured by the CSO Participatory Environment Index. Decentralization captures local offices' relative power (A) and whether the executive/legislature is locally elected (B). The solid line indicates the interaction of health aid and social engagement at mean levels of decentralization. Weakly decentralized countries are indicated by the short-dashed line (reflecting one standard deviation below the mean). Strongly decentralized countries are indicated by the long-dashed line (reflecting one standard deviation above the mean). Health aid (DAH) is lagged by one period.

population health, even with substantial health aid per capita and an engaged citizenry. Conversely, recipient countries like Guinea in the late 1990s, where local office holders are appointed rather than locally elected and lack autonomous decision-making, experienced increased health aid effectiveness alongside high social engagement. Specifically in Guinea, moderate levels of health aid combined with an engaged citizenry led to an annual decrease in infant mortality by about 3.5 percent, despite the country's centralized governance. This pattern suggests the benefits of social engagement are more pronounced in centralized countries where local offices hold limited power and are primarily appointed rather than locally elected. This finding contradicts Hypothesis 4a and implies that political and administrative decentralization weakens, rather than strengthens, the positive impact of social engagement.

Figure 6.6 replicates this finding for political engagement. In particular, each plot (A–D) demonstrates that rising elite-entrusting political engagement enhances aid effectiveness predominantly in centralized rather than decentralized settings. The enhancing effect of a politically engaged citizenry is most pronounced when local and regional governments hold limited power (A and B), when local officials are appointed rather than elected, and when subnational governments have little authority over taxing, spending, and legislation (D). Conversely, in decentralized countries with quasi-autonomous, locally elected subnational governments, rising political engagement does not foster aid effectiveness. This result is replicated across different model specifications and alternative decentralization measures, as detailed in table A6.8 and table A6.9. In sum, the reported evidence suggests that decentralization does not strengthen the enhancing effect of elite-entrusting political engagement, contradicting Hypothesis 4b.

Decentralization and Elite-Challenging Engagement

An open question is how decentralization impacts contentious, elite-challenging forms of political engagement. In theory, locally elected officials with decision-making and administrative authority should be more responsive to citizen demands from elite-challenging actions, as decentralization tightens the accountability loop between providers and users of public services. To examine whether the observed synergistic effect of elite-challenging mass movements is larger in decentralized countries, population health is regressed on decentralization, health aid, and their interactions with citizen participation in mass movements, as detailed in table 6.6.

The reported estimates and the significant three-way interaction term imply that decentralization strengthens the enhancing impact of citizen action for accountability. This highlights the importance of decentralization, particularly for elite-challenging as opposed to elite-entrusting modes of civic engagement. Figure 6.7 visualizes this interaction, displaying the marginal effect of health aid across observed levels of citizen protest and decentralization. For both pro-democratic and anti-system movements, the figure demonstrates that the enhancing impact of contentious political engagement on aid effectiveness is significantly stronger in decentralized countries. Specifically, in recipient countries with locally elected legislative and executive offices and quasi-autonomous local governments, increased elite-challenging action enhances health aid effectiveness. This is indicated

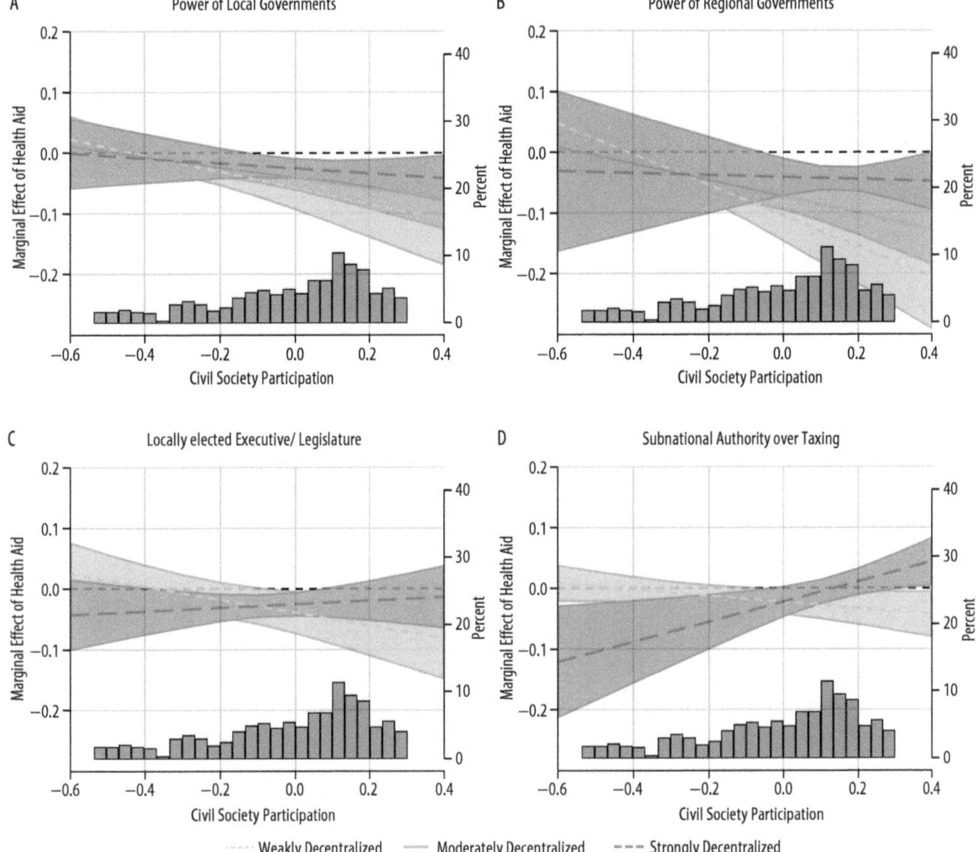

Figure 6.6. Political Engagement, Decentralization, and the Marginal Effect of Health Aid. *Note:* Figure shows average marginal effects of lagged health aid on infant mortality across the observed range of political engagement and at different levels of decentralization. Plots A–D visualize the estimates of Models 4–7 reported in table 6.5. Political engagement is measured by the Civil Society Participation index. Decentralization is measured by the relative power of local governments (A) and regional governments (B), whether the executive/legislature is locally elected (C), and whether subnational governments have authority over taxing, spending, and legislation (D). The solid line indicates the interaction of health aid and political engagement at mean levels of decentralization. Weakly decentralized countries are indicated by the short-dashed line (reflecting one standard deviation below the mean/non-decentralized countries). Strongly decentralized countries are indicated by the long-dashed line (reflecting one standard deviation above the mean/decentralized countries). Health aid (DAH) is lagged by one period.

Table 6.6. Elite-Challenging Action, Decentralization, and Health Aid Effectiveness

	Dependent Variable: Infant Mortality Rate (Log Scale)							
	Panel 1: Anti-System Movements				Panel 2: Pro-Democratic Movements			
	Regional Government Elected		Locally Elected Executive/ Legislature		Power of Local Governments		Locally Elected Executive/ Legislature	
	(1)	(2)	(3)	(4)	(5)	(6)	(7)	(8)
DAH (log scale)	−0.021*	−0.027***	0.001	−0.014	−0.007	−0.011	−0.001	−0.001
	(0.012)	(0.009)	(0.015)	(0.030)	(0.008)	(0.008)	(0.015)	(0.028)
Elite-challenging action	−0.007	−0.008	0.015	0.011	0.019	0.020	0.014	0.016
	(0.013)	(0.012)	(0.021)	(0.022)	(0.014)	(0.013)	(0.017)	(0.021)
DAH (log scale) * Elite-challenging action	−0.000	−0.005	0.025	0.018	−0.005	−0.009	0.009	0.004
	(0.011)	(0.008)	(0.020)	(0.017)	(0.008)	(0.007)	(0.009)	(0.010)
Decentralization	0.011	0.010	−0.057	−0.000	0.020	0.025*	−0.021	0.016
	(0.011)	(0.009)	(0.035)	(0.046)	(0.014)	(0.013)	(0.034)	(0.027)
DAH (log scale) * Decentralization	−0.003	0.001	−0.021	−0.015	−0.009	−0.008	−0.001	−0.005
	(0.007)	(0.008)	(0.020)	(0.031)	(0.007)	(0.007)	(0.018)	(0.028)
Elite-challenging action * Decentralization	−0.007	−0.004	−0.008	−0.008	0.008	0.009	0.022	0.002
	(0.008)	(0.008)	(0.026)	(0.036)	(0.009)	(0.008)	(0.026)	(0.025)
DAH (log scale) * Elite-challenging action * Decentralization	−0.018**	−0.014**	−0.062***	−0.044**	−0.012*	−0.012*	−0.027*	−0.018*
	(0.008)	(0.006)	(0.021)	(0.018)	(0.006)	(0.006)	(0.016)	(0.010)
IMR (lagged)	1.093***	1.067***	1.095***	1.040***	1.049***	1.035***	1.062***	1.058***
	(0.027)	(0.029)	(0.034)	(0.064)	(0.044)	(0.044)	(0.036)	(0.047)

	Dependent Variable: Infant Mortality Rate (Log Scale)							
	Panel 1: Anti-System Movements				Panel 2: Pro-Democratic Movements			
	Regional Government Elected		Locally Elected Executive/ Legislature		Power of Local Governments		Locally Elected Executive/ Legislature	
	(1)	(2)	(3)	(4)	(5)	(6)	(7)	(8)
Constant	−0.238	0.000	0.000	0.000	0.000	−0.268	−0.912***	0.000
	(0.219)	(0.000)	(0.000)	(0.000)	(0.000)	(0.332)	(0.291)	(0.000)
Basic controls	Yes	Yes	Yes	Yes	Yes	Yes	Yes	Yes
Public−sector corruption	Yes	Yes	Yes	Yes	Yes	Yes	Yes	Yes
Fertility rate (log scale)		Yes				Yes	Yes	Yes
Female education				Yes				
Physicians (log scale)							Yes	Yes
HIV prevalence (log scale)								Yes
Observations	409	409	374	305	325	325	268	207
Countries	107	107	99	80	97	97	82	62
Instruments	95	104	95	103	104	113	113	113
Hansen−test	0.375	0.471	0.406	0.972	0.478	0.645	0.987	1
AR2	0.122	0.118	0.321	0.631	0.639	0.653	0.693	0.775

Note: Table shows two-step GMM estimation with Windmeijer bias-corrected robust standard errors. Elite-challenging action is measured by the Anti-System Movements (Models 1–4) and the Pro-Democratic Movements (Models 5–8) indices. Health aid (DAH) is lagged by one period. Decentralization captures local governments' relative power and whether local or regional offices of the executive or legislature are locally elected. Basic controls include period fixed effects, conflict involvement, GDP per capita (log scale), and population size (log scale). DAH, elite-challenging action, and decentralization are mean-centered. *** $p < 0.01$, ** $p < 0.05$, * $p < 0.1$.

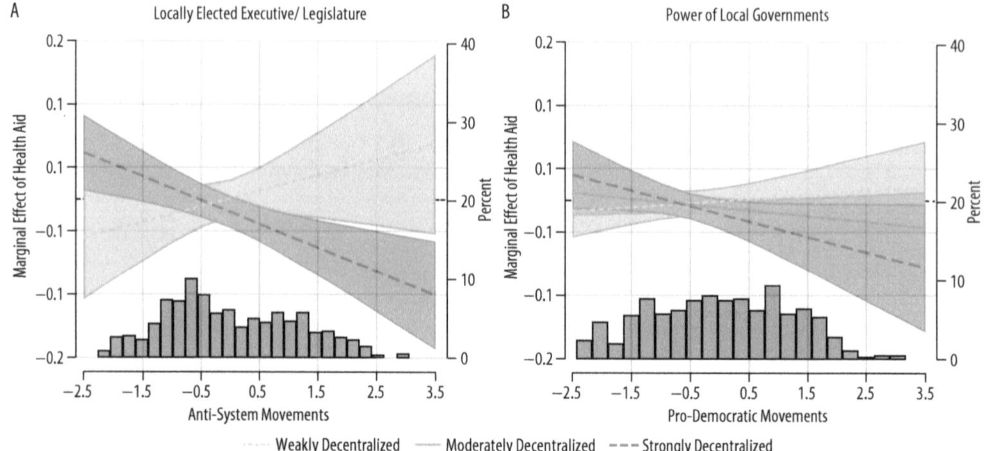

Figure 6.7. Elite-Challenging Action, Decentralization, and the Marginal Effect of Health Aid. *Note:* Figure shows average marginal effects of lagged health aid on infant mortality across the observed range of elite-challenging action and at different levels of decentralization. Elite-challenging action is measured as Anti-System Movements (A) and Pro-Democratic Movements (B) based on Models 3 and 6 in table 6.6. Decentralization reflects whether the executive/legislature is locally elected or not (A) and the relative power of local governments (B). The solid line indicates the interaction of health aid and political engagement at mean levels of decentralization. Weakly decentralized countries are indicated by the short-dashed line (reflecting one standard deviation below the mean/non-decentralized countries). Strongly decentralized countries are indicated by the long-dashed line (reflecting one standard deviation above the mean/decentralized countries). Health aid (DAH) is lagged by one period.

by the negatively sloped long-dashed marginal effect lines in both plots (A and B). For instance, in the late 1990s, politically active citizens engaging in mass accountability actions enabled Mexico's autonomous local governments to convert international health funding into an annual decline in infant mortality of above 5 percent. But in less or moderately decentralized recipient countries, such as Cameroon in the early 1990s, the effects of health aid along varying levels of citizen protest fail to be statistically significant or even change sign, decreasing population health. By implication, decentralization fosters the enhancing impact of engaged citizens participating in elite-challenging actions. This finding remains robust across alternative model specifications and after controlling for differences in state capacity (table A6.10). In brief, bringing governments "closer" to the people strengthens the enhancing impact of elite-challenging political engagement on the effectiveness of health aid.

To summarize, there is little evidence suggesting that political or administrative decentralization strengthens the enhancing effect of social and elite-entrusting political engagement. Neither does the transfer of authority from the central to the local level directly enhance health aid effectiveness. Rather, health aid tends to be most effective in centralized recipient countries with a vibrant voluntary sector and an engaged, noncontentious civil society. Conversely, in decentralized countries with autonomous, locally elected officials, increased citizen engagement fails to enhance aid effectiveness. This implies that decentralization undermines the enhancing effects of social engagement and elite-entrusting political participation, contradicting Hypotheses 4a and 4b.

This finding echoes evidence from political economy studies, suggesting that ill-defined mandates and responsibilities between central and local authorities impede coordination and cooperation in the provision of public services (Lessmann and Markwardt 2012). It is also in line with recent evidence on the effects of federalism on US health policy, particularly its impact on citizens' political attitudes and actions, perpetuating political disempowerment among low-income citizens (Michener 2018). Nevertheless, in the context of elite-challenging accountability action, decentralization does strengthen the observed relationship between political engagement and health aid effectiveness, aligning with Hypothesis 4c. Thus, health aid proves most effective when citizens seek accountability through elite-challenging activities and local officials face clear, formally institutionalized incentives to respond. Conversely, in centrally organized recipient countries, rising contentious political engagement can entirely offset the benefits of health aid. In other words, elite-challenging actions make development assistance for health work best in decentralized countries where locally elected officials are equipped with the administrative and decision-making authority to respond to citizen demands.

Summary

The previous chapter showed that health aid is more effective in countries where citizens regularly attend community meetings, participate in political and non-political civil-society organizations, and demand accountability through elite-challenging action. This chapter examined whether formal institutions of bureaucratic governance, democratic oversight, and decentralization strengthen the identified enhancing effects of civic engagement. Two key findings emerge: First, social and elite-entrusting political engagement enhances health aid effectiveness regardless of political context. A vibrant voluntary sector and a politically active citizenry can make health aid more effective even in the most corrupt, undemocratic, and centralized recipient country. Second, in contrast, elite-challenging political engagement boosts health aid effectiveness most prominently in bureaucratic, democratic, and decentralized states. Consequently, citizen participation in elite-challenging actions makes health aid work best in recipient countries with strong (1) administrative and organizational capacities, (2) democratic oversight institutions, and (3) decentralized administrative and decision-making authority.

1. Regarding bureaucratic governance, the evidence suggests that state capacity strengthens the enhancing effects of elite-challenging actions but not of social and noncontentious political engagement. Thus, citizen action for accountability has the largest impact on aid effectiveness when recipient governments have greater capacities to respond to citizen demands. Citizen participation in voluntary activities, community work, and political associations enhances aid effectiveness, however, even in recipient countries with dysfunctional state institutions. Elite-entrusting forms of citizen engagement are thus functionally equivalent to strong state institutions and foster the effectiveness of health aid even in countries where states lack decision-making and organizational capacity.

2. Similarly, democratic oversight institutions strengthen the enhancing effect of elite-challenging mass movements but do not change the impact of elite-entrusting forms of citizen engagement. In recipient countries that guarantee democratic rights, increased demand for accountability through elite-challenging action makes health aid more effective. By contrast, under authoritarian rule, rising elite-challenging activities fail to increase health aid effectiveness. The lack of democratic institutions thus undermines the aid effectiveness enhancing impact of citizen action for accountability. Yet the quality

of democracy does not influence the effects of social and elite-entrusting political engagement, which can make aid work better even in the least democratic environments. Hence, despite dysfunctional democratic oversight institutions, a vibrant voluntary sector and a politically active citizenry beyond mass movements can enhance health aid effectiveness.

3. Lastly, administrative and political decentralization fosters mass movements' impact on aid effectiveness but undermines the enhancing effects of social and elite-entrusting political engagement. In particular, the transfer of power and authority to the local level in recipient countries strengthens the synergistic impact of elite-challenging action on making aid more effective. Mass movements thus make health aid most effective in recipient countries with strongly decentralized authorities. Yet reducing the distance between governments and citizens undermines the enhancing effects of elite-entrusting forms of civic engagement. In particular, the more administrative authority is centrally organized, the more a vibrant voluntary sector and citizen engagement in political matters make aid work. In other words, social and elite-entrusting political engagement enhances the effectiveness of health aid, particularly in recipient countries with firmly centralized authorities.

Analyzing the political context conditions of citizen engagement in recipient countries has shown it is essential to distinguish between elite-entrusting and elite-challenging modes of citizen participation. Elite-entrusting forms of social and political engagement foster the effectiveness of health aid primarily in recipient countries with weak formal institutions. But elite-challenging modes of participation only strengthen the effects of aid on public health if top-down mechanisms of performance oversight ensure accountability through democratic institutions, an organizational structure in which bureaucracies exert control based on standard operating procedures and meritocratic recruitment, and the transfer of power and responsibility from central to local authorities. Hence, bureaucratic governance, liberal democracy, and decentralization of authority to subnational levels constitute enabling conditions under which elite-challenging actions make a positive difference in health aid effectiveness.

NOTES

1. If bureaucratic governance is measured by a country's level of corruption control, we would expect a significant *positive* three-way interaction term because state fragility is inversely related to state capacity and corruption control.

2. Table A6.1 and table A6.2 in the appendix report additional robustness checks on the combined effect of health aid and political engagement based on V-Dem's Participatory Component index and Civil Society Participation index, respectively, in the context of varying levels of state fragility.

3. This finding is confirmed when using alternative indices for social engagement and political engagement, as reported in table A6.5.

4. Chapter 5 directly compares the moderating effect of social engagement with the conditioning role of democratic institutions (table A5.13). The evidence shows a significant interaction between health aid and social engagement and an insignificant interaction between health aid and democratic institutions for each of the different measures of top-down oversight mechanisms.

5. The Freedom House Political Rights subindex measures the presence of free elections, political pluralism, and the functioning of government, while the Civil Liberties subindex measures freedom of expression and belief, associational and organizational rights, the rule of law, and autonomy and individual rights.

6. The short-dashed marginal effect line shows the estimated effect of health aid on infant mortality for undemocratic recipient countries as proxied by one standard deviation below the average level of liberal democracy. The long-dashed marginal effect line shows the estimated effect of health aid on infant mortality for democratic recipient countries as proxied by one standard deviation above the average level of liberal democracy. The solid marginal effect line indicates the interaction of health aid and elite-challenging action at moderate levels of liberal democracy.

Why Civic Engagement Matters

The positive relationship between civic engagement and citizen action for accountability is a well-established finding in political culture research. Yet its implications for the effectiveness of development assistance have not been tested on a comparative basis. Existing literature emphasizes the role of formal institutions and "good governance" in determining the effectiveness of foreign aid (Chauvet 2015; Wright and Winters 2010). Meanwhile, donors have shifted the focus of development interventions from capacity development to strengthening civic engagement and beneficiary participation, empowering civil-society organizations to acquire the necessary information, resources, and capacities to monitor and evaluate development outcomes and hold public officials accountable (O'Neil, Foresti, and Hudson 2007). At the same time, donors placed more emphasis on strengthening recipients' health systems, and development assistance for health saw a significant increase in absolute and relative terms. Evidence on the effectiveness of health interventions remains inconclusive, however, resulting from the failure to recognize that health systems are social institutions shaped by community relations. Furthermore, the macro-comparative aid effectiveness literature has entirely ignored the role of citizen action for accountability despite consensus on the developmental and democratizing effects of citizen engagement.

Closing this gap and expanding previous research, this study has focused on cultural and political factors shaping accountability in public-service delivery and asked whether ordinary people make development assistance for health work better. I have argued that health aid is more effective in recipient countries with a socially and politically engaged citizenry. The reason is that citizen engagement fosters communities' willingness and capacity to voice shared concerns and exercise pressure to hold public authorities and organizational providers accountable and engage in participatory health projects. I have further argued that formal institutions of bureaucratic governance, democratic oversight, and decentralization determine the strength of the enhancing effects of civic engagement by creating incentives that influence citizen demand and government responsiveness. This book thus draws attention to the growing understanding of health systems as social institutions that operate through the various relationships between ordinary people and different health-system actors (Sheikh, Ranson, and Gilson 2014).

The theoretical propositions were tested in three steps. The first part of the empirical analysis tested the widely held belief that voluntary organizations instill value orientations that strengthen individuals' willingness to keep elites honest, accountable, and responsive to citizens' needs, and that they provide a training ground for the development of civic skills that foster communities' capacity to engage in oversight activities and citizen-led accountability action.

The analysis revealed that citizen engagement in voluntary organizations is associated with higher interest in community affairs, stronger norms of cooperation, greater support for liberal democracy, and value orientations that emphasize freedom of choice, equal opportunities, and citizen voice. This general finding must be qualified because members of religious organizations differ regarding their liberal social attitudes and democratic orientations, although they are also more interested in community affairs and equally share norms of civic cooperation. The evidence further suggests that citizen involvement, including religious engagement, increases citizens' participation in elite-challenging mass movements. These results support the claim that people who join political and non-political voluntary associations are more willing and better able to voice shared concerns and exercise pressure on public officials and service providers. Social and political engagement thus empowers ordinary people in aid recipient countries to demand accountability and participate in oversight activities.

Resting on a broader data basis, these findings disprove claims from social-capital research that associational involvement suppresses elite-challenging action and supports the stability of authoritarian regimes (Roßteutscher 2010; Jamal 2009). Instead, social and political engagement strengthens citizen demand for accountability across various regions and institutional contexts. This finding approves Western donors' efforts to empower ordinary people to demand accountability and oversee donor programs.

Based on the established link between citizen engagement and demand for accountability, the second part of the empirical analysis addressed the central question of whether health aid is more effective in countries with higher social and political engagement. The results of a dynamic panel study indicate that citizen engagement is an important determinant of health aid effectiveness. Hence, development assistance for health reduces infant mortality more effectively in recipient countries where citizens frequently participate in voluntary activities or unpaid community work and engage in elite-challenging actions. In other words, ordinary people who regularly attend community meetings and are active in diverse civil-society organizations make health aid work better. These results are robust to accounting for endogeneity and selection bias.

The magnitude of the estimated effects is substantial. Health aid allocated to recipient countries with an active citizenry that has the capacity to hold governments accountable is more than twice as effective in reducing infant mortality compared to an average recipient country. In fact, given that donors tend to allocate more health aid to fragile countries that are less likely to achieve progress in population health (Graves, Haakenstad, and Dieleman 2015), the reported effects of health aid are likely to be conservative estimates.[1] Furthermore, comparing the effects of civic engagement with the impact of formal accountability mechanisms demonstrates that state capacity and democratic institutions do not significantly enhance the effectiveness of health aid after controlling for citizen involvement. This finding underlines the importance of citizen engagement over formally institutionalized mechanisms and, thus, the advantage of bottom-up over top-down processes of performance oversight in making aid work better.

Evidence from a multilevel study proves that an active citizenry also strengthens health aid effectiveness at the individual level. Specifically, citizen engagement in voluntary associations that pursue social and political interests, excluding faith-based organizations, makes health aid increase individuals' self-rated health status. Comparing the role of social and political engagement demonstrates that participation in political and professional organizations has the strongest enhancing effect on making health aid work. The individual-level evidence establishes the micro-foundation of the identified ecological interaction pattern between civic engagement and health aid. Overall, both studies lend strong support for the proposed synergistic effects of social and political engagement on the effectiveness of health aid. These findings complement existing qualitative evidence on the democratic and developmental outcomes of citizen engagement in voluntary associations and citizen-led social accountability actions. According to this evidence, civic engagement enhances knowledge and awareness of entitlements, fosters a sense of agency and empowerment, and increases communities' capacity to demand accountability (Gaventa and Barrett 2012; Joshi 2013). The findings also generalize evidence on the essential role of community-based organizations in the provision of health services, including HIV-related prevention, care, and treatment (Nair et al. 2010; Riehman et al. 2013; Campbell et al. 2013; David and Li 2010).

The third part of this study re-examined the role of civic engagement and further explored the institutional conditions under which social and political engagement makes health aid work. In doing so, it examined to what extent the enhancing impact of civic engagement depends on specific political contexts that enable citizens to demand accountability and cause governments to respond to citizens' preferences. The study focused on a set of institutional factors that arguably strengthen the effects of citizen involvement, including strong state institutions, democratic oversight institutions, and the decentralization of administrative and decision-making authority.

The relevance of the formal political context is based on the following considerations. Bureaucratic governance reflects the ability of a state to maintain control and political sovereignty within the borders of its territory and to expand public welfare and prosperity. Based on standard operating procedures and meritocratic recruitment promoting competence over loyalty, bureaucratic governance ensures that decision-making authority rests in the office and not in the person of the incumbent. Higher technical and managerial capacity should enable strong bureaucratic states to respond to citizen demands by setting and communicating health system priorities, carrying out health policies, and monitoring their achievement. Decision-making and organizational competence, in turn, shape citizen expectations about government responsiveness and thus influence individuals' motivation to engage in costly accountability actions. Democratic institutions should strengthen accountability and government responsiveness mainly by enabling an independent judiciary and legislature to prosecute illegal behavior and impose formal sanctions based on citizen complaints and grievances. Democratic oversight mechanisms were thus expected to bolster the impact of civic engagement on aid effectiveness. Additionally, decentralizing authority from the central to the local level was hypothesized to foster the impact of citizen engagement by giving service users a real say in the planning and implementation of development interventions and by creating incentives for local officials to respond to those they are supposed to serve and by whom they are elected.

Against this backdrop, the third part tested whether formal institutions of bureaucratic governance, democratic oversight, and decentralization foster the observed synergistic impact of civic engagement. The study revealed two main findings. First, higher state capacity, democratic quality, and the transfer of power and responsibility to the local level do not strengthen the enhancing effects of social and elite-entrusting political engagement. In fact, the influence of elite-entrusting citizen participation on higher aid effectiveness is strongest in recipient countries where formal institutions are weak or absent. Thus, a vibrant voluntary sector and a politically active citizenry can make health aid work better even in patronage, authoritarian, and centralized recipient countries.

Yet, second, the political context plays a major role when it comes to elite-challenging political engagement. While citizen protest under average context conditions increases aid effectiveness, the enhancing effects of elite-challenging activities are largest under established bureaucratic governance, liberal democracy, and decentralization. Thus, citizen participation in elite-challenging action makes health aid most effective in recipient countries with strong decision-making and organizational capacities, democratic oversight institutions, and decentralized administrative and decision-making authority.

With regard to bureaucratic governance, the study's findings imply that social-movement activities enhance health aid effectiveness if states are able to maintain social order and security and have the decision-making and organizational competence to respond to increased citizen demands. Thus, state institutions that promote competence over loyalty and exert control based on the principles of impartiality, efficiency, transparency, and integrity determine whether or not citizen-led accountability action fosters the effectiveness of health aid. This finding resonates with evidence from social-accountability studies demonstrating that citizen engagement is more effective when bolstered by high state capacity, supporting the claim that "voice needs teeth to have a bite—but teeth may not bite without voice" (Fox 2015, 357). Likewise, it is consistent with evidence from social-movement research demonstrating that elite-challenging action is more likely to be violent if a state lacks the capacity to respond to citizen demands (Tilly 2006; Tilly and Tarrow 2015).

Conversely, the outcomes of elite-entrusting forms of civic engagement do not depend on high state capacity. Thus, citizen involvement in voluntary organizations and community activities can make health aid work without functional state institutions. In fact, citizen participation in voluntary activities, community work, and political associations enhances the effectiveness of health aid even in fragile recipient countries with rampant corruption—thus, where it is most needed. Yet, in bureaucratic states that have the decision-making capacity and organizational competence to expand public welfare, increased elite-entrusting civic engagement contributes little to improved health aid effectiveness. This result suggests that, on the one hand, elite-entrusting citizen engagement can substitute dysfunctional state institutions and make health aid work better. On the other hand, elite-entrusting civic engagement loses its enhancing effect in the context of a bureaucratic state that is able to implement public-health decisions with the appropriate organizational means and is less dependent on coproduction by users and communities.

These findings echo evidence from comparative research on areas of limited statehood (Börzel and Risse 2016). This literature shows that the effective provision of public goods and services does not necessarily depend on a strong central authority but can also rely on generalized trust emerging from personal ties in local communities. Evidence from this literature also suggests that engagement in local associations does not necessarily undermine citizen support for a central government but may rather enhance the stability of a state in the long run (Murtazashvili 2016).

Regarding the quality of democracy, existing literature highlights the importance of independent oversight institutions authorized to impose formal sanctions in response to citizen demands. Yet this study finds no indication that democratic institutions support the synergistic effects of elite-entrusting citizen engagement. Even in the least democratic context, social and particularly political engagement can make health aid work better.

Democratic institutions significantly influence the impact of elite-challenging political engagement on health aid effectiveness, however. Under democratic rule, citizen protest enhances the effectiveness of health aid, whereas, under authoritarian rule, it undermines the positive effect of aid on population health. In other words, whether citizen protest enhances the effectiveness of health development interventions depends on the presence of democratic oversight institutions.

The findings resonate with the propositions of selectorate theory on the interplay between democratic governance, citizen protest, and the source of government revenue (Bueno de Mesquita and Smith 2009; 2010). This theory posits that in undemocratic recipient countries, political leaders misappropriate non-tax revenues, like foreign aid, to reduce the threat from elite-challenging mass movements. Consequently, the enhancing impact of elite-challenging activities diminishes when large-scale citizen action poses a threat to the stability of the political system, and basic democratic institutions are absent. The findings are also consistent with more recent conceptualizations of the developmental state (Evans and Heller 2015) and insights from social-movement research indicating that elite-challenging actions are less violent if democratic institutions guarantee civic space and provide protection from arbitrary action by governmental agents such as police, judges, and public officials (Tilly and Tarrow 2015, 57).

Concerning the role of decentralization, existing literature suggests that lowering the distance between governments and citizens enables users to better monitor service delivery and incentivizes providers to respond to local demands. This study reveals that the devolution of power to local authorities in recipient countries has differential effects on the impact of elite-challenging and elite-entrusting forms of citizen engagement. Specifically, while decentralization weakens the enhancing impact of elite-entrusting civic engagement, it strengthens those of elite-challenging engagement. Consequently, centralized administrative authorities and responsibilities strengthen the enhancing impact of social and elite-entrusting political engagement on aid effectiveness. In decentralized recipient countries with quasi-autonomous, locally elected officials, however, increased social and political engagement fails to enhance health aid effectiveness. This suggests that decentralization weakens the synergistic effects of elite-entrusting civic engagement because of coordination challenges between central and local authorities and the influence of local power elites, who have little interest in improving public-service delivery (Prud'homme 1995; Bardhan 2002). Recent studies further corroborate this finding by highlighting how federalism shapes citizen's experiences with health-care providers and undermines communities' capacity to engage in politics (Michener 2018).

Yet, in decentralized recipient countries where citizens regularly engage in social movements and protests, this study finds that health aid is more effective. Specifically, development assistance has a more positive effect on public health when locally elected, autonomous officials have the administrative and decision-making authority to respond to citizen demands through elite-challenging action. This suggests that when local officials face institutional incentives to respond to local demands, health aid effectiveness benefits from increased political engagement. These findings resonate with studies highlighting the advantages of transferring health services to local governments that have some discretion and are downwardly accountable (Mansuri and Rao 2013, 8) and with research from fragile states where local associations effectively collaborate with district-level officials (Murtazashvili 2016, 245–255).

In conclusion, this study provides robust evidence that development assistance is linked to better health outcomes if widespread social and political participation empowers citizens to hold public authorities accountable and directly engage in participatory development projects. The quantitative approach adopted here generalizes this finding across different context conditions and complements existing case studies and experimental evidence. Thereby, this study not only provides macro-comparative evidence but also examines the impact of civic engagement and aid on individuals' subjective health status based on multilevel analyses. The study design accounts for a set of health-related individual characteristics, including age, education, and income, and eliminates differences linked to the political and socioeconomic context. The consistent results of the panel data and multilevel analyses thus provide robust evidence about the cultural and political conditions that make health aid work better at the macro and the individual level. Furthermore, the use of data from various sources, including international public-opinion surveys and expert ratings, demonstrates that the results obtained are consistent for different social and political engagement measures. The empirical analysis therefore provides robust evidence across different units of analysis and samples of recipient countries, supporting the relationship proposed by the theory.

Given that health aid is only one among different sources of development financing, it is worth noting that controlling for domestic public-health expenditures or non-health-related development assistance leads to qualitatively similar results and does not alter the identified enhancing effects of civic engagement.[2] The evidence also suggests that aid allocated to other sectors such as education, environmental protection, civil society, or agriculture differs from health aid as it is neither directly nor indirectly (conditionally) associated with population health. These considerations support the former conclusion that the health aid effects reported in this study are unlikely to be biased and underline donors' commitment to strengthen civic engagement.

Future research will benefit from the increased availability of subnational and geocoded data on development projects and health policies, offering insights into the links between civic engagement, policy outputs, and aid effectiveness beyond the national level. It will shed light on the variation in civic engagement within countries and help scholars determine whether local civic capacity enhances the effectiveness of local development interventions. Furthermore, it will help to better understand the distributional effects of aid, as people who benefit most from participatory development interventions tend to be better educated, more engaged, and less geographically isolated (Mansuri and Rao 2013, 6).

Improved data availability will also strengthen the reliability of estimation strategies accounting for endogeneity issues. This study applied different quantitative estimation techniques, including GMM estimation and Heckman's two-stage selection models, to adequately model the dynamics and interactions between determinants of population health. These techniques control for the simultaneity of the aid allocation and aid effectiveness process and take into account non-aid recipient countries to avoid selectivity bias. While most tests on the validity of the instrumentation strategy are passed comfortably, larger panels and longer time series will enable future research to specify different dynamics and strengthen the reliability of GMM estimates.

To fully comprehend the implications of the findings reported in this study, future research will have to extend the analysis beyond the health sector. Additional macro-comparative investigations are necessary to ascertain whether similar positive impacts arise from the interaction of civic engagement with other sector-specific aid. Broadening the research focus will enhance our understanding of the multifaceted benefits of an engaged citizenry and allow donors to allocate resources across sectors more effectively.

Wrapping It Up and Policy Implications

Civic engagement is both a means and an end to effective development assistance. Despite its importance, the existing aid effectiveness literature has entirely overlooked the role of civic engagement and demand-side mechanisms of accountability. Expanding previous research, this study explores the cultural and political conditions under which development assistance for health reduces poverty, paying particular attention to the coordination challenges that prevent citizens in aid recipient countries from holding officials and providers accountable.

The reported evidence demonstrates that a vibrant voluntary sector and a politically active citizenry that engages with public officials and mobilizes political action make health-development interventions more effective even in recipient countries with dysfunctional formal institutions. Specifically, citizen engagement in voluntary associations and social movements cultivates politically interested individuals who are motivated and able to keep those involved in development processes honest, accountable, and responsive to their needs. Civic engagement thus makes citizens more likely to participate in accountability actions and to engage with service providers and public officials in aid recipient countries. It also determines citizens' direct involvement in development projects that provide space for beneficiary engagement linked to the design, monitoring, and evaluation of development interventions. These relationships help explain why development assistance for health has been more effective in recipient countries with weak formal accountability mechanisms but active citizenries. Ordinary citizens can thus make an important contribution to building responsive states that provide better access to services, and to translating civil-society activity into developmental improvements.

These findings have important implications for donors and policymakers seeking to make development interventions more effective. The most important implication is the need to understand that recipients' health systems are social institutions shaped by community relations, norms of co-operation, and value orientations that are embedded in different political contexts. It requires health-development interventions to be sensitive to the local setting, including a country's history, and to acknowledge the complex interactions between cultural and political factors (Carothers 2011, 342–344).

On the one hand, taking into account the local context of recipient countries implies designing culturally responsive programs that consider how context shapes motivation for action. Development interventions often rely on models of agency and the self that reflect the culture of independence prevalent in most Western donor countries. In contrast, many recipient countries are characterized by a culture of interdependence (Thomas and Markus 2023). Thus, considering the cultural differences between independent donor and interdependent recipient countries in styles of motivation, behavioral drivers, and relational forces can help better align development programs with the needs of target populations (Thomas and Markus 2023, 205–206). For instance, development interventions can foster community over individual empowerment approaches and emphasize interdependent motives and values in program communications, such as social responsibility and community collaboration. Moreover, the effectiveness of interventions can be enhanced by considering the social obligations and relational forces that shape the preferences of communities for selecting beneficiaries of a development program and, as a result, the legitimacy of different targeting approaches among community members. Donors should also place more emphasis on understanding what motivates citizens to engage as agents of social change and what determines their development priorities (Han 2009). For example, putting development priorities into context implies acknowledging differences in what is perceived as the most pressing public-health issue and aligning the objectives of development interventions accordingly (Badaan and Choucair 2023, 239–240).

On the other hand, taking into account cultural and political contexts requires paying more attention to the organizational landscape in recipient countries and how communities overcome collective-action dilemmas in the absence of formal institutions rather than engaging in fruitless attempts of state building (Börzel and Risse 2016; Murtazashvili 2016). Strengthening communities' motivation and capacity to engage in collective action requires supporting the whole associational ecosystem in recipient countries, including the private sector, which has often been a significant driver of change (Van Rooy 2013). Less-visible community associations and those representing the interests of marginalized groups (e.g., women's associations) require special attention to even out the unequal power distribution among citizens (Grandvoinnet, Aslam, and Raha 2015).

Additionally, strengthening inter-group relationships and networks for collective action is crucial in bridging social and ethnic divides among recipient communities. This implies supporting activities that help to build vertical and horizontal links among civil-society actors at the local and national levels and between professionalized and membership-based organizations (Anderson, Fox, and Gaventa 2020). It also involves helping civic organizations maintain the trust of their members by supporting them to diversify their sources of revenue and ensure their financial autonomy and independence from donor interests (Edwards 2020, 122–124). It further implies bringing elites on board as allies in the empowerment of the poor, including cooperating with traditional and religious leaders (Grandvoinnet, Aslam, and Raha 2015). Therefore, establishing public spaces that facilitate dialogue and discussion is essential, specifically by promoting free and independent media involving community radio. A pluralistic media landscape is crucial not only in maintaining public scrutiny and raising awareness of rights and entitlements but also in disseminating information about aid programs and increasing transparency to ensure that citizens actively participate and benefit from aid.

Even though civic engagement can improve health aid effectiveness in fragile states, there are also risks, especially when citizens engage in regime-threatening forms of political action. Specifically, under authoritarian rule, aid is likely to be diverted away from its intended purposes to lower the threat of regime collapse if a significant share of the citizenry is engaged in elite-challenging action. Increased elite-challenging political participation can thus reduce the quality of public-good provision if formal institutions of democratic governance are absent. Equally, elite-challenging actions also weaken the effectiveness of aid-funded service delivery in weak and centralized states that lack the organizational capacity and the decision-making authority to respond to citizen demands. So, in corrupt, undemocratic, and centralized recipient countries, increased mass actions for accountability weaken the effectiveness of donor-funded public-health interventions.

Conversely, in recipient countries with an independent judiciary and legislature that can prosecute illegal behavior, these social movements and citizen protests improve health service delivery. Citizen engagement in elite-challenging actions also enhances the effectiveness of donor-funded health services in bureaucratic states that have the organizational capacities to maintain social order and in decentralized states where power and authority are transferred to locally elected officials that are more open to public scrutiny and face incentives to respond to local demands. Hence, elite-challenging actions make health aid most effective in countries with strong decision-making and organizational capacities, democratic oversight institutions, and decentralized governance.

The observed effects of citizen participation in elite-entrusting and elite-challenging activities are consistent with findings from citizen-engagement studies. For instance, Gaventa and Barrett found that while social movements can increase state responsiveness, in less democratic contexts, citizen engagement in local associations rather than social movements is far more important in holding authorities accountable (2012, 2404–2406). Similarly, evidence from social-movement research highlights the role of democratic institutions in guaranteeing space for citizen action and the state's capacity to respond to citizen demands (Tilly and Tarrow 2015, 56–58). This body of evidence suggests that in high-capacity democratic environments, social movements are less violent, while weak state capacity increases the likelihood of violent social movements with adverse effects on population health (Tilly 2006, 81).

These insights have significant implications for donors and policymakers aiming to reduce poverty in violent and fragile settings. Generally speaking, donors should seek to protect spaces for citizens to voice their claims, monitor state reprisals, and promote citizen action for accountability. This includes protecting the right to association, ensuring universal access to political participation, and strengthening formal processes of participatory governance. Such efforts expand civil society's watchdog function and enable citizens to channel their preferences into decision-making and activate mechanisms of legal accountability. In fragile contexts, however, opportunities for accountability actions are often limited. Furthermore, deferent attitudes to authorities, fear of repression, and distrust prevent many citizens from participating in community affairs (Joshi 2023). Donors should, therefore, concentrate on interventions that create safe spaces for organizations to collaborate, build trust and social capital, and overcome the fear of engaging with authorities, particularly at the local level (Gaventa and Oswald 2019; Gaventa, Joshi, and Anderson 2023). Moreover, they should be present in multiple locations and support the horizontal spread and coordination of coalitions of actors rather than single actors that are more vulnerable to targeting by the authorities (Gaventa and Oswald 2019, 11). This involves collaborating with networks and alliances that engage in human-rights activities and provide legal and human-rights support (Anderson et al. 2022). Donors working in challenging contexts may also decide to reduce public visibility in recipient countries and use less politically charged language in project reports to avoid authoritarian governments being suspicious of foreign funding and undermining the legitimacy of civil-society actors (Tadros 2020).

It is also important to recognize the role of trigger events, which provide opportunities for change and can unleash more complex forms of contention (Gaventa 2023). For instance, given that women play a significant role in mobilizing elite-challenging action, donors can concentrate on supporting social movements that focus on gender-based discrimination and repressive gender norms, thereby providing important entry points for women to become organized and involved in politics (Gaventa, Joshi, and Anderson 2023, 8; Anderson, Fox, and Gaventa 2020, Carothers 2011, 345). Thus, instead of directly supporting movements around "democracy," focusing on collective mobilization around less contentious issues can have positive spillover effects on empowerment and accountability demands.[3]

Furthermore, donors should simultaneously coordinate citizen voice initiatives with reforms that build the capacity of institutions to respond to increased citizen demands (Fox 2015; Carothers 2011, 342–344; Gaventa and Oswald 2019). Such multilevel approaches focus on vertically aggregating information on citizens' preferences and experiences with local service providers to national policy debates, integrating citizen demands into the activities of different advocacy networks, and building coalitions of pro-accountability forces within and across multiple localities and sectors to prevent the fragmentation of civil society (Anderson, Fox, and Gaventa 2020, 31). Multilevel approaches provide important entry points for donors who work in fragile and conflict-affected contexts and seek to strengthen accountability.

In conclusion, understanding the organizational landscape in recipient countries and the role of civic engagement is essential for informed policy design and for the future study of aid effectiveness. Donors should concentrate on supporting the emergence of collective action and strengthening associational life and inter-group relationships. A particular focus on the empowerment of women is vital to broaden citizen demands for accountability, particularly in fragile and challenging political environments. Taking cultural context seriously also implies refining the design and implementation of development interventions and avoiding overly simplistic assumptions of citizens' motivation to engage in accountability actions.

NOTES

1. The reason is that omitting an unobserved factor that positively determines aid allocation and negatively affects population health tends to mask rather than exaggerate health aid effectiveness.

2. Theoretically, development assistance to any sector may relax government budget constraints because of the fungibility of aid and ultimately influence health outcomes. For instance, funding for water supply and sanitation, waste management, and domestic government health expenditures are likely to improve population health. Similarly, development interventions that foster education can indirectly improve health outcomes. Under the assumption that increased aid to non-health sectors or domestic expenditures "crowd in" development assistance for health, not accounting for these effects could theoretically inflate estimates of health aid effectiveness.

3. Given that social movements mobilize actions that increase the odds of democratic transition, donor efforts to strengthen civic participation indirectly create the institutional conditions under which elite-challenging action makes health aid work better. Therefore, on the one hand, strengthening civic engagement improves the effects of health aid on population health by increasing citizen demand for accountability in service delivery. On the other hand, civic engagement helps create a legal and political space for citizens to engage in political actions that are found to make health aid more effective.

Acknowledgments

Every book embarks on a unique journey. This one has taken a long and winding one, with invaluable contributions from people to whom I owe many debts of gratitude. Foremost, my heartfelt thanks go to my wife and family for their unwavering belief in me and my work. This book is dedicated to you. To my friends, I am deeply grateful for the companionship and enriching conversations that have made this journey a truly memorable one.

Over the years, I have had the privilege of working with remarkable colleagues and students at Leuphana University Lüneburg from whom I have learned a great deal. I am particularly indebted to Christian Welzel for his invaluable mentorship that shaped my thinking about political behavior and development. I am also immensely grateful to Ferdinand Müller-Rommel for his ongoing professional support during my time at the Center for the Study of Democracy. Many colleagues lent their expertise to this project. In particular, I thank Amy C. Alexander, Steven Brieger, Lennart Brunkert, Björn Buß, Cristina Carbonell Betancourt, Franziska Deutsch, Feit Ebermann, Dawid Friedrich, Vera van Hüllen, Marcus Kronfeldt, Tim Kunkowski, Maria Ravlik, Michelangelo Vercesi, Lena Wach, and Nina-Kathrin Wienkoop. This book also owes immense debts to my former colleagues at the Hamburg Institute of International Economics, who shared their thoughts on initial ideas or read through draft chapters, including Andre Wolf, Meike Löhr, Lars Wenzel, and Henrik Harms. Special acknowledgment goes to Jörg Faust from the German Institute for Development Evaluation for his valuable feedback, and Robert Franzese for technical support at the ICPSR Summer Program 2019 at the University of Michigan. I am grateful to Antje Reuleke, Hannes Harnack, Anna Saave, Jonathan Fox, Matthew S. Winters, Ruth Carlitz, Gabriella Montinola, and three anonymous reviewers for their valuable feedback. I would also like to thank the FAZIT Foundation for supporting this project, and my editor at Johns Hopkins University Press, Robin Coleman, for his continuous encouragement.

References

Acht, Martin, Toman Omar Mahmoud, and Rainer Thiele. 2014. "Corrupt Governments Receive Less State-to-State Aid: Governance and the Delivery of Foreign Aid Through Non-State Actors." *Journal of Development Economics* 114: 20–33.

Addison, Tony, Oliver Morrissey, and Finn Tarp. 2017. "The Macroeconomics of Aid: Overview." *Journal of Development Studies* 53 (7): 987–997.

Afridi, Muhammad Asim, and Bruno Ventelou. 2013. "Impact of Health Aid in Developing Countries: The Public vs. the Private Channels." *Economic Modelling* 31 (1): 759–765.

Ahlerup, Pelle, Ola Olsson, and David Yanagizawa. 2009. "Social Capital vs Institutions in the Growth Process." *European Journal of Political Economy* 25 (1): 1–14.

AidData. 2017. "AidDataCore_ResearchRelease_Level1_v3.1 Research Releases Dataset." AidData (website). Accessed February 20, 2020. https://www.aiddata.org/data/aiddata-core-research-release-level-1-3-1.

Aiken, Leona S., and Stephen G. West. 1991. *Multiple Regression: Testing and Interpreting Interactions*. London: SAGE Publications Ltd.

Ajzen, I. 2012. "The Theory of Planned Behavior." In *Handbook of Theories of Social Psychology*, vol. 1, edited by P. A. M. Lange, A. W. Kruglanski, and E. T. Higgins. London: SAGE Publications Ltd.

Alagappa, Muthiah. 2004. *Civil Society and Political Change in Asia: Expanding and Contracting Democratic Space*. Stanford: Stanford University Press.

Almond, Gabriel Abraham, and Sidney Verba. 1963. *The Civic Culture: Political Attitudes and Democracy in Five Nations*. London: SAGE Publications Ltd.

Alvarez, Melisa Martínez, and Arnab Acharya. 2012. "Effectiveness in the Health Sector." UNU-WIDER Working Paper no. 2012/69, United Nations University World Institute for Development Economics Research, Helsinki.

Anderson, Colin, Jonathan Fox, and John Gaventa. 2020. "How Do Donor-Led Empowerment and Accountability Activities Take Scale into Account? Evidence from DFID Programmes in Contexts of Fragility, Conflict and Violence." IDS Working Paper 536, Institute of Development Studies, Brighton, UK.

Anderson, Colin, John Gaventa, Jenny Edwards, Anuradha Joshi, N. J. Nampoothiri, and Emily Wilson. 2022. "Against the Odds: Action for Empowerment and Accountability in Challenging Contexts." A4EA Policy and Practice Paper, Institute of Development Studies, Brighton, UK.

Anderson, Colin, Anuradha Joshi, Katrina Barnes, et al. 2023. "Everyday Governance in Areas of Contested Power: Insights from Mozambique, Myanmar, and Pakistan." *Development Policy Review* 41 (S1): 1–18.

Andrews, Matt. 2013. *The Limits of Institutional Reform in Development: Changing Rules for Realistic Behaviour*. Cambridge, UK: Cambridge University Press.

Andrews, Rhys. 2012. "Social Capital and Public Service Performance: A Review of the Evidence." *Public Policy and Administration* 27: 49–67.

Anheier, Helmut, and Jeremy Kendall. 2002. "Interpersonal Trust and Voluntary Associations: Examining Three Approaches." *British Journal of Sociology* 53 (3): 343–362.

Ardic, Nurullah. 2012. "Understanding the 'Arab Spring': Justice, Dignity, Religion and International Politics." *Afro Eurasian Studies* 1 (1): 8–52.

Armony, Ariel. 2004. *The Dubious Link: Civic Engagement and Democratization.* Stanford, CA: Stanford University Press.

Arnall, Alex, David S. G. Thomas, Chasca Twyman, and Diana Liverman. 2013. "NGOs, Elite Capture and Community-Driven Development: Perspectives in Rural Mozambique." *Journal of Modern African Studies* 51 (2): 305–330.

Arndt, Channing, Sam Jones, and Finn Tarp. 2015. "Assessing Foreign Aid's Long Run Contribution to Growth and Development." *World Development* 69: 6–18.

Arugay, Aries A. 2016. "Sanctions, Rewards and Learning: Enforcing Democratic Accountability in the Delivery of Health, Education, and Water, Sanitation and Hygiene." International IDEA Discussion Paper no. 16/2016, International Institute for Democracy and Electoral Assistance, Stockholm.

Auer, Benjamin, and Horst Rottmann. 2011. *Statistik und Ökonometrie für Wirtschaftswissenschaftler.* 2nd ed. Wiesbaden: Gabler Verlag.

Badaan, Vivienne, and Farah Choucair. 2023. "Toward Culturally Sensitive Development Paradigms: New Shifts, Limitations, and the Role of (Cross-) Cultural Psychology." *Journal of Cross-Cultural Psychology* 54 (2): 232–248.

Baguley, Thom. 2012. *Serious Stats: A Guide to Advanced Statistics for the Behavioral Sciences.* New York: Palgrave Macmillan.

Baiocchi, Gianpaola. 2003. "Participation, Activism, and Politics: The Porto Alegre Experiment." In *Deepening Democracy: Institutional Innovations in Empowered Participatory Governance,* edited by Archon Fung and Erik Olin Wright. London: Verso.

Baliamoune-Lutz, Mina. 2012. "Do Institutions and Social Cohesion Enhance the Effectiveness of Aid? New Evidence from Africa." *Journal of International Commerce, Economics and Policy* 3 (1): 1–19.

Baliamoune-Lutz, Mina, and George Mavrotas. 2009. "Aid Effectiveness: Looking at the Aid-Social Capital-Growth Nexus." *Review of Development Economics* 13 (3): 510–525.

Baltagi, Badi H. 2005. *Econometric Analysis of Panel Data.* 3rd ed. Chichester, UK: Wiley.

Banerjee, Abhijit, Rukmini Banerji, Esther Duflo, Rachel Glennerster, and Stuti Khemani. 2010. "Pitfalls of Participatory Programs: Evidence from a Randomized Evaluation in Education in India." *American Economic Journal: Economic Policy* 2 (1): 1–30.

Banks, Arthur. 2015. Cross-National Time-Series Data Archive (CNTS). State University of New York at Binghamton. https://www.cntsdata.com.

Banks, Nicola, David Hulme, and Michael Edwards. 2015. "NGOs, States, and Donors Revisited: Still Too Close for Comfort?" *World Development* 66: 707–718.

Bano, Masooda. 2012. *Breakdown in Pakistan: How Aid Is Eroding Institutions for Collective Action.* Stanford, CA: Stanford University Press.

Bardhan, Pranab. 2002. "Decentralization of Governance and Development." *Journal of Economic Perspectives* 16 (4):185–205.

Bardhan, Pranab, and Dilip Mookherjee. 2006. "Decentralisation and Accountability in Infrastructure Delivery in Developing Countries." *Economic Journal* 116 (508): 101–127.

Baskaran, Thushyanthan, Arne Bigsten, and Zohal Hessami. 2013. "Political Decentralization and the Effectiveness of Aid." In *Globalization and Development: Rethinking Interventions and Governance*, edited by Arne Bigsten. New York: Routledge.

Bauer, Daniel J., and Patrick J. Curran. 2005. "Probing Interactions in Fixed and Multilevel Regression: Inferential and Graphical Techniques." *Multivariate Behavioral Research* 40 (3): 373–400.

Beck, Nathaniel, and Jonathan N. Katz. 2011. "Modeling Dynamics in Time-Series-Cross-Section Political Economy Data." *Annual Review of Political Science* 14 (1): 331–352.

Beck, Thorsten, George Clarke, Alberto Groff, Philip Keefer, and Patrick Walsh. 2001. "New Tools in Comparative Political Economy: The Database of Political Institutions." *World Bank Economic Review* 15 (1):165–176.

Bendavid, Eran, and Jay Bhattacharya. 2009. "The President's Emergency Plan for AIDS Relief in Africa: An Evaluation of Outcomes." *Annals of Internal Medicine* 150 (10): 688–695.

Bendavid, Eran, and Jay Bhattacharya. 2014. "The Relationship of Health Aid to Population Health Improvements." *JAMA Internal Medicine* 174 (6): 881–887.

Bendavid, Eran, Charles B. Holmes, Jay Bhattacharya, and Grant Miller. 2012. "HIV Development Assistance and Adult Mortality in Africa." *JAMA: The Journal of the American Medical Association* 307 (19): 2060–2067.

Bennett, Sara. 2011. "Health System Strengthening: Past, Present and Future." In *Routledge Handbook of Global Public Health*, edited by Richard Parker and Marni Sommer. New York: Routledge.

Berger, Ben. 2009. "Political Theory, Political Science and the End of Civic Engagement." *Perspectives on Politics* 7 (2): 335.

Berman, Sheri. 1997. "Civil Society and Political Institutionalization." *American Behavioral Scientist* 40 (5): 562–574.

Bermeo, Sarah Blodgett. 2011. "Foreign Aid and Regime Change: A Role for Donor Intent." *World Development* 39 (11): 2021–2031.

Bernhard, Michael, Dong Joon Jung, Eitan Tzelgov, Michael Coppedge, and Staffan I. Lindberg. 2017. "Making Embedded Knowledge Transparent: How the V-Dem Dataset Opens New Vistas in Civil Society Research." *Perspectives on Politics* 15 (2): 342–360.

Berry, William D., Matt Golder, and Daniel Milton. 2012. "Improving Tests of Theories Positing Interaction." *Journal of Politics* 74 (3): 653–671.

Birn, Anne-Emanuelle, Yogan Pillay, Timothy H. Holtz, and Paul F. Basch. 2009. *Textbook of International Health: Global Health in a Dynamic World*. 3rd ed. Oxford: Oxford University Press.

Björkman, Martina, and Jakob Svensson. 2009. "Power to the People: Evidence from a Randomized Field Experiment on Community-Based Monitoring in Uganda." *Quarterly Journal of Economics* 124 (2): 735–769.

Björkman Nyqvist, Martina, Damien de Walque, and Jakob Svensson. 2017. "Information Is Power: Experimental Evidence on the Long-Run Impact of Community Based Monitoring." *American Economic Journal: Applied Economics* 9 (1): 33–69.

Bjørnskov, Christian. 2010. "How Does Social Trust Lead to Better Governance? An Attempt to Separate Electoral and Bureaucratic Mechanisms." *Public Choice* 144: 323–346.

Blair, Harry. 2000. "Participation and Accountability at the Periphery: Democratic Local Governance in Six Countries." *World Development* 28 (1): 21–39.

Blair, Harry. 2011. "Gaining State Support for Social Accountability." In *Accountability Through Public Opinion: From Inertia to Public Action*, edited by Sina Odugbemi and Taeku Lee. Washington DC: World Bank.

Bliss, Frank. 2009. "Partizipation in der Entwicklungsplanung: Anspruch und Wirklichkeit." *Aus Politik und Zeitgeschiche* 34–35: 20–26.

Blomkvist, Hans, and Katrin Uba. 2010. "Civil Society and Social Capital in South Asia." In *International Encyclopedia of Civil Society*, edited by Helmut Anheier and Stefan Toepler. New York: Springer.

Blundell, Richard, and Stephen Bond. 1998. "Initial Conditions and Moment Restrictions in Dynamic Panel Data Models." *Journal of Econometrics* 87 (1): 115–143.

Boix, Carles, and Daniel N. Posner. 1996. "Making Social Capital Work: A Review of Robert Putnam's Making Democracy Work: Civic Traditions in Modern Italy." Working Paper no. 96-4, Weatherhead Center for International Affairs, Harvard University.

Boone, Peter. 1996. "Politics and the Effectiveness of Foreign Aid." *European Economic Review* 40 (2): 289–329.

Booth, John A., and Patricia Bayer Richard. 1998. "Civil Society, Political Capital, and Democratization in Central America." *Journal of Politics* 60 (3): 780–800.

Börzel, Tanja A., and Thomas Risse. 2010. "Governance Without a State: Can It Work?" *Regulation and Governance* 4 (2): 113–134.

Börzel, Tanja A., and Thomas Risse. 2016. "Dysfunctional State Institutions, Trust, and Governance in Areas of Limited Statehood." *Regulation & Governance* 10: 149–160.

Boulding, Carew. 2014. *NGOs, Civil Society, and Political Protest*. New York: Cambridge University Press.

Bourdieu, Pierre. 1983. "Ökonomisches Kapital, Kulturelles Kapital, Soziales Kapital." In *Soziale Ungleichheiten*, special edition, edited by Reinhard Kreckel. Göttingen: Soziale Welt.

Bourdieu, Pierre. 1986. "The Forms of Capital." In *Handbook of Theory and Research for the Sociology of Education*, edited by John G. Richardson. New York: Greenwood.

Bourguignon, François, and Mark Sundberg. 2007. "Is Foreign Aid Helping? Aid Effectiveness—Opening the Black Box." *American Economic Review* 97 (2): 316–321.

Brady, Henry E., Sidney Verba, and Kay Lehman Schlozman. 1995. "Beyond SES: A Resource Model of Political Participation." *American Political Science Review* 89 (2): 271–294.

Brambor, Thomas, William Roberts Clark, and Matt Golder. 2006. "Understanding Interaction Models: Improving Empirical Analyses." *Political Analysis* 14 (1): 63–82.

Bratton, Michael, Robert Mattes, and E. Gyimah-Boadi. 2004. *Public Opinion, Democracy, and Market Reform in Africa*. Cambridge, UK: Cambridge University Press.

Bräutigam, Deborah A., and Stephen Knack. 2004. "Foreign Aid, Institutions, and Governance in Sub-Saharan Africa." *Economic Development and Cultural Change* 52 (2): 255–285.

Brett, E. A. 2003. "Participation and Accountability in Development Management." *Journal of Development Studies* 40 (2): 1–29.

Brinkerhoff, Derick W., and Anna Wetterberg. 2013. "Performance-Based Public Management Reforms: Experience and Emerging Lessons from Service Delivery Improvement in Indonesia." *International Review of Administrative Sciences* 79 (3): 433–457.

Brinkerhoff, Derick W., and Anna Wetterberg. 2016. "Gauging the Effects of Social Accountability on Services, Governance, and Citizen Empowerment." *Public Administration Review* 76 (2): 274–286.

BTI. 2014. Bertelsmann Transformation Index. *Paraguay Country Report.* Gütersloh: Bertelsmann Stiftung.

Bueno de Mesquita, Bruce, James D. Morrow, Randolph M. Siverson, and Alastair Smith. 2002. "Political Institutions, Policy Choice and the Survival of Leaders." *British Journal of Political Science* 32 (4): 559–590.

Bueno de Mesquita, Bruce, and Alastair Smith. 2009. "Political Survival and Endogenous Institutional Change." *Comparative Political Studies* 42 (2): 167–197.

Bueno de Mesquita, Bruce, and Alastair Smith. 2010. "Leader Survival, Revolutions, and the Nature of Government Finance." *American Journal of Political Science* 54 (4): 936–950.

Bueno de Mesquita, Bruce, Alastair Smith, Randolph M. Siverson, and James D. Morrow. 2003. *The Logic of Political Survival.* Cambridge, MA: MIT Press.

Buntaine, Mark T., and Bradley Parks. 2013. "When Do Environmentally Focused Assistance Projects Achieve Their Objectives?" *Global Environmental Politics* 13 (2): 65–88.

Burnside, Craig, and David Dollar. 2000. "Aid, Policies, and Growth." *American Economic Review* 90 (4): 847–868.

Burnside, Craig, and David Dollar. 2004. "Aid, Policies and Growth: Revisiting the Evidence." World Bank Policy Research Working Paper 3251, Washington, DC.

Burzynska, Katarzyna, and Olle Berggren. 2015. "The Impact of Social Beliefs on Microfinance Performance." *Journal of International Development* 277 (7): 1074–1097.

Busse, Matthias, and Steffen Gröning. 2009. "Does Foreign Aid Improve Governance?" *Economics Letters* 104 (2): 76–78.

Cameron, Adrian Colin, and Pravin Trivedi. 2009. *Microeconometrics Using Stata.* College Station, TX: Stata Press.

Campbell, Catherine, Kerry Scott, Mercy Nhamo, et al. 2013. "Social Capital and HIV Competent Communities: The Role of Community Groups in Managing HIV/AIDS in Rural Zimbabwe." *AIDS Care* 25 (Suppl. 1): S114–S122.

Carey, John M., and Matthew Soberg Shugart. 1995. "Incentives to Cultivate a Personal Vote: A Rank Ordering of Electoral Formulas." *Electoral Studies* 14 (4): 417–439.

Carlitz, Ruth. 2013. "Improving Transparency and Accountability in the Budget Process: An Assessment of Recent Initiatives." *Development Policy Review* 31 (S1): 49–67.

Carothers, Thomas. 2011. *Aiding Democracy Abroad: The Learning Curve.* Washington DC: Carnegie Endowment for International Peace.

Castiglione, Dario. 2008a. "Introduction: Conceptual Issues in Social Capital Theory." In *The Handbook of Social Capital*, edited by Dario Castiglione, Jan van Deth, and Guglielmo Wolleb. New York: Oxford University Press.

Castiglione, Dario. 2008b. "Introduction: Social Capital Between Community and Society." In *The Handbook of Social Capital*, edited by Dario Castiglione, Jan van Deth, and Guglielmo Wolleb. New York: Oxford University Press.

Castiglione, Dario. 2008c. "Social Capital as a Research Programme." In *The Handbook of Social Capital*, edited by Dario Castiglione, Jan van Deth, and Guglielmo Wolleb. New York: Oxford University Press.

Charron, Nicholas. 2011. "Exploring the Impact of Foreign Aid on Corruption: Has the 'Anti-Corruption Movement' Been Effective?" *Developing Economies* 49 (1): 66–88.

Chauvet, Lisa. 2015. "On the Heterogenous Impact of Aid on Growth: A Review of the Evidence." In *Handbook on the Economics of Foreign Aid*, edited by Mak Arvin and Byron Lew. Cheltenham, UK: Edward Elgar Publishing.

Chauvet, Lisa, Flore Gubert, and Sandrine Mesplé-Somps. 2013. "Aid, Remittances, Medical Brain Drain and Child Mortality: Evidence Using Inter and Intra-Country Data." *Journal of Development Studies* 49 (6): 801–818.

Cheibub, José Antonio, Jennifer Gandhi, and James Raymond Vreeland. 2010. "Democracy and Dictatorship Revisited." *Public Choice* 143 (1): 67–101.

Cleary, Susan M., Sassy Molyneux, and Lucy Gilson. 2013. "Resources, Attitudes and Culture: An Understanding of the Factors That Influence the Functioning of Accountability Mechanisms in Primary Health Care Settings." *BMC Health Services Research* 13: 320.

Cohen, Jacob, Patrici Cohen, Stephen G. West, and Leona S. Aiken. 2003. *Applied Multiple Regression/Correlation Analysis for the Behavioral Sciences*. 3rd ed. London: Lawrence Erlbaum Associates.

Coleman, James. 1988. "Social Capital in the Creation of Human Capital." *American Journal of Sociology* 94 (1988): 95–120.

Coleman, James. 1990. *Foundations of Social Theory*. Cambridge, MA: Harvard University Press.

Collier, Paul, and David Dollar. 2002. "Aid Allocation and Poverty Reduction." *European Economic Review* 46 (8): 1475–1500.

Coppedge, Michael, John Gerring, Carl Henrik Knutsen, et al. 2019. "V-Dem Codebook v9." Varieties of Democracy (V-Dem) Project, Varieties of Democracy Institute, Gothenburg, Sweden.

Coppedge, Michael, John Gerring, Carl Henrik Knutsen, et al. 2020. "V-Dem Codebook v10." Varieties of Democracy (V-Dem) Project, Varieties of Democracy Institute, Gothenburg, Sweden.

Cornwall, Andrea. 2006. "Historical Perspectives on Participation in Development." *Commonwealth and Comparative Politics* 44 (1): 62–83.

Cornwall, Andrea. 2008. "Unpacking 'Participation' Models, Meanings and Practices." *Community Development Journal* 43 (3): 269–283.

Cornwall, Andrea, and Vera Schattan Coelho, eds. 2007. *Spaces for Change: The Politics of Citizen Participation in New Democratic Arenas*. London: Zed Books.

DAC. 2008. "Is It ODA? Factsheet." Development Assistance Committee (DAC) OECD Publishing. Accessed December 28, 2017. http://www.oecd.org/dac/stats/34086975 .pdf (page discontinued).

DAC. 2009. "Glossar Entwicklungspolitischer Schlüsselbegriffe aus den Bereichen Evaluierung und Ergebnisorientiertes Management." Development Assistance Committee (DAC) OECD Publishing.

DAC. 2012. "Development Co-operation Report 2012: Lessons in Linking Sustainability and Development." Development Assistance Committee (DAC) OECD Publishing. https://doi.org/10.1787/dcr-2012-en.

DAC. 2016. "Development Aid at a Glance. Statistics by Region. Developing Countries." 2016. Accessed April 21, 2017. http://www.oecd.org/dac/stats /documentupload/World-Development-Aid-at-a-Glance.pdf (page discontinued).

Dalgaard, Carl-Johan, and Henrik Hansen. 2001. "On Aid, Growth and Good Policies." *Journal of Development Studies* 37 (6): 17–41.

Dalgaard, Carl-Johan, and Henrik Hansen. 2009. "Evaluating Aid Effectiveness in the Aggregate: Methodological Issues." *Evaluation Study 2009/1*. Copenhagen: Ministry of Foreign Affairs of Denmark. Danida's Evaluation Department.

Dalgaard, Carl-Johan, and Henrik Hansen. 2010. "Evaluating Aid Effectiveness in the Aggregate: A Critical Assessment of the Evidence." *Evaluation Study 2010/1*. Copenhagen: Ministry of Foreign Affairs of Denmark. Danida's Evaluation Department.

Dalgaard, Carl-Johan, Henrik Hansen, and Finn Tarp. 2004. "On the Empirics of Foreign Aid and Growth." *Economic Journal* 114 (496): F191–F216.

Dasgupta, Aniruddha, and Victoria A. Beard. 2007. "Community Driven Development, Collective Action and Elite Capture in Indonesia." *Development and Change* 38 (2): 229–249.

David, Antonio C., and Carmen A. Li. 2010. "Exploring the Links between HIV/AIDS, Social Capital, and Development." *Journal of International Development* 22 (7): 941–961. https://doi.org/10.1002/jid.1707.

De Jongh, Thyra E., Joanne H. Harnmeijer, Rifat Atun, et al. 2014. "Health Impact of External Funding for HIV, Tuberculosis and Malaria: Systematic Review." *Health Policy and Planning* 29 (5): 650–662.

De Renzio, Paolo. 2005. "Scaling Up Versus Absorptive Capacity: Challenges and Opportunitites for Reaching the MDGs in Africa." ODI Briefing Paper, Overseas Development Institute, London.

De Renzio, Paolo, Vitus Azeem, and Vivek Ramkumar. 2006. "Budget Monitoring as an Advocacy Tool: Lessons from Civil Society Budget Analysis and Advocacy Initiatives." Uganda Debt Network Case Study, Uganda Debt Network.

Diamond, Larry. 1999. *Developing Democracy: Toward Consolidation*. Baltimore: Johns Hopkins University Press.

Dieleman, Joseph L., Casey Graves, and Michael Hanlon. 2013. "The Fungibility of Health Aid: Reconsidering the Reconsidered." *Journal of Development Studies* 49 (12): 1755–1762.

Dieleman, Joseph L., Casey Graves, Elizabeth Johnson, et al. 2015. "Sources and Focus of Health Development Assistance, 1990–2014." *JAMA* 313 (23): 2359–2368.

Dietrich, Simone. 2011. "The Politics of Public Health Aid: Why Corrupt Governments Have Incentives to Implement Aid Effectively." *World Development* 39 (1): 55–63.

Dietrich, Simone, and Joseph Wright. 2013. "Foreign Aid and Democratic Development in Africa." In *Democratic Trajectories in Africa*, edited by Danielle Resnick and Nicolas Van de Walle. Oxford: Oxford University Press.

Dijkstra, Geske. 2013. "The New Aid Paradigm: A Case of Policy Incoherence." DESA Working Paper no. 128, UN World Economic and Social Survey.

Djankov, Simeon, Jose G. Montalvo, and Marta Reynal-Querol. 2008. "The Curse of Aid." *Journal of Economic Growth* 13 (3): 169–194.

Dodds, Anneliese. 2012. *Comparative Public Policy*. Basingstoke, UK: Palgrave Macmillan.

Dollar, David, and Victora Levin. 2005. "Sowing and Reaping: Institutional Quality and Project Outcomes in Developing Countries." World Bank Policy Research Working Paper 3524, Washington, DC.

Dorsner, Claire. 2004. "Social Exclusion and Participation in Community Development Projects: Evidence from Senegal." *Social Policy & Administration* 38 (4): 366–382.

Draude, Anke, Tanja A. Börzel, and Thomas Risse, eds. 2018. *The Oxford Handbook of Governance and Limited Statehood*. Oxford: Oxford University Press.

Dramé, Fatou Maria, Emily E. Crawford, Daouda Diouf, Chris Beyrer, and Stefan D. Baral. 2013. "A Pilot Cohort Study to Assess the Feasibility of HIV Prevention Science Research Among Men Who Have Sex with Men in Dakar, Senegal." *Journal of the International AIDS Society* 16 (Suppl. 3): 18742–18903.

Drèze, Jean, and Amartyá Sen. 1995. *India: Economic Development and Social Opportunity*. Oxford: Oxford University Press.

Duber, Herbert C., Thomas J. Coates, Greg Szekeras, Amy H. Kaji, and Roger J. Lewis. 2010. "Is There an Association Between PEPFAR Funding and Improvement in National Health Indicators in Africa? A Retrospective Study." *Journal of the International AIDS Society* 13 (21): 1–9.

Durlauf, Steven N., and Marcel Fafchamps. 2004. "Empirical Studies of Social Capital: A Critical Survey." NBER Working Paper Series no. 10485, National Bureau of Economic Research, Cambridge, MA.

Dwicaksono, Adenantera, and Ashley M. Fox. 2018. "Does Decentralization Improve Health System Performance and Outcomes in Low- and Middle-Income Countries? A Systematic Review of Evidence from Quantitative Studies." *Milbank Quarterly* 96 (2): 323–368.

Dyson, Tim. 2013. "On Demographic and Democratic Transitions." *Population and Development Review* 38: 83–102.

Easterly, William. 2003. "Can Foreign Aid Buy Growth?" *Journal of Economic Perspectives* 17 (3): 23–48.

Easterly, William. 2007. "Are Aid Agencies Improving?" *Economic Policy* 22 (52): 633–678.

Easterly, William, ed. 2008. *Reinventing Foreign Aid*. Cambridge, MA: MIT Press.

Eckstein, Harry, and Ted Robert Gurr. 1975. *Patterns of Authority: A Structural Basis for Political Inquiry*. New York: John Wiley & Sons Inc.

Edwards, Bob, and Michael W. Foley. 2001. "Civil Society and Social Capital: A Primer." In *Beyond Tocqueville: Civil Society and the Social Capital Debate in Comparative Perspective*, edited by Bob Edwards, Michael W. Foley, and Mario Diani. Hanover, NH: University Press of New England.

Edwards, Michael. 2020. *Civil Society*. 4th ed. Cambridge, UK: Polity Press.

Edwards, Michael, and David Hulme. 1996. "Too Close for Comfort? The Impact of Official Aid on Nongovernmental Organizations." *World Development* 24 (6): 961–973.

Eggen, Øyvind, and Kjell Roland. 2013. *Western Aid at a Crossroads: The End of Paternalism*. Basingstoke, UK: Palgrave Pivot.

Esser, Hartmut. 2008. "The Two Meanings of Social Capital." In *The Handbook of Social Capital*, edited by Dario Castiglione, Jan van Deth, and Guglielmo Wolleb. New York: Oxford University Press.

Evans, Peter, and Patrick Heller. 2015. "Human Development, State Transformation, and the Politics of the Developmental State." In *The Oxford Handbook of Transformations of the State*, edited by Stephan Leibfried, Evelyne Huber, Matthew Lange, Jonah D. Levy, Frank Nullmeyer, and John D. Stephens. Oxford: Oxford University Press.

Evans, Peter B., and James E. Rauch. 1999. "Bureaucracy and Growth: A Cross-National Analysis of the Effects of 'Weberian' State Structures on Economic Growth." *American Sociological Review* 64 (5): 748–765.

Evans, Peter B., Dietrich Rueschemeyer, and Theda Skocpol, eds. 1985. *Bringing the State Back In*. Cambridge, UK: Cambridge University Press.

Faguet, Jean-Paul. 2014. "Decentralization and Governance." *World Development* 53: 2–13.

Falleti, Tulia G., and Santiago L. Cunial. 2018. *Participation in Social Policy: Public Health in Comparative Perspective*. Cambridge, UK: Cambridge University Press.

Farag, Marwa, A. K. Nandakumar, Stanley Wallack, Dominic Hodgkin, Gary Gaumer, and Can Erbil. 2013. "Health Expenditures, Health Outcomes and the Role of Good Governance." *International Journal of Health Care Finance and Economics* 13 (1): 33–52.

Fielding, David. 2011. "Health Aid and Governance in Developing Countries." *Health Economics* 20 (7): 757–769.

Fielding, David, and Stephen Knowles. 2011. "Dangerous Interactions: Problems in Interpreting Tests of Conditional Aid Effectiveness." *World Economy* 34 (6): 972–983.

Finsterbusch, Kurt, and Warren A. Van Wicklin. 1987. "The Contribution of Beneficiary Participation to Development Project Effectiveness." *Public Administration and Development* 7: 1–23.

Finsterbusch, Kurt, and Warren A. Van Wicklin. 1989. "Beneficiary Participation in Development Projects: Empirical Tests of Popular Theories." *Economic Development and Cultural Change* 37 (3): 573–593.

Flaxman, Abraham D., Nancy Fullman, Mac W. Otten, et al. 2010. "Rapid Scaling Up of Insecticide-Treated Bed Net Coverage in Africa and Its Relationship with Development Assistance for Health: A Systematic Synthesis of Supply, Distribution, and Household Survey Data." *PLoS Medicine* 7 (8): 1–17.

Foa, Roberto, and Grzegorz Ekiert. 2017. "The Weakness of Postcommunist Civil Society Reassessed." *European Journal of Political Research* 56 (2): 419–439.

Foa, Roberto, and Jeffery Tanner. 2012. "Methodology of the Indices of Social Development." ISD Working Paper 2012-4, The Hague.

Foley, Michael W., and Bob Edwards. 1996. "The Paradox of Civil Society." *Journal of Democracy* 7 (3): 38–52.

Fox, Jonathan. 2015. "Social Accountability: What Does the Evidence Really Say?" *World Development* 72: 346–361.

Freitag, Markus, and Paul C. Bauer. 2013. "Testing for Measurement Equivalence in Surveys: Dimensions of Social Trust Across Cultural Contexts." *Public Opinion Quarterly* 77 (S1): 24–44.

Fukuyama, Francis. 2004. *State-Building, Governance and World Order in the 21st Century.* Ithaca, NY: Cornell University Press.

Fung, Archon. 2003. "Associations and Democracy: Between Theories, Hopes, and Realities." *Annual Review of Sociology* 29 (1): 515–539.

Fung, Archon, and Erik Olin Wright. 2003. "Thinking About Empowered Participatory Governance." In *Deepening Democracy: Institutional Innovations in Empowered Participatory Governance*, edited by Archon Fung and Erik Olin Wright. London: Verso.

Gakidou, Emmanuela, Krycia Cowling, Rafael Lozano, and Christopher Murray. 2010. "Increased Educational Attainment and Its Effect on Child Mortality in 175 Countries Between 1970 and 2009: A Systematic Analysis." *Lancet* 376: 959–974.

Gaventa, John. 2023. "Repertoires of Citizen Action in Hybrid Settings." *Development Policy Review* 41 (S1).

Gaventa, John, and Gregory Barrett. 2012. "Mapping the Outcomes of Citizen Engagement." *World Development* 40 (12): 2399–2410.

Gaventa, John, Anuradha Joshi, and Colin Anderson. 2023. "Citizen Action for Accountability in Challenging Contexts: What Have We Learned?" *Development Policy Review* 41 (S1): 1–17.

Gaventa, John, and Rosemary McGee. 2010. *Citizen Action and National Policy Reform: Making Change Happen.* Edited by John Gaventa and Rosemary McGee. London: Zed Books.

Gaventa, John, and Katy Oswald. 2019. *Empowerment and Accountability in Difficult Settings: What Are We Learning?* Brighton, UK: IDS.

Genschel, Philipp, and Bernhard Zangl. 2014. "State Transformations in OECD Countries." *Annual Review of Political Science* 17: 337–354.

Gerring, John, Carl Henrik Knutsen, and Jonas Berge. 2022. "Does Democracy Matter?" *Annual Review of Political Science* 25: 357–375.

Gerring, John, Strom C. Thacker, and Rodrigo Alfaro. 2012. "Democracy and Human Development." *Journal of Politics* 74 (1): 1–17.

Gibson, Clark C., Krister Andersson, Elinor Ostrom, and Sujai Shivakumar. 2005. *The Samaritan's Dilemma: The Political Economy of Development Aid.* Oxford: Oxford University Press.

Gilbert, Leah. 2010. "Civil Society and Social Capital in Russia." In *International Encyclopedia of Civil Society*, edited by Helmut Anheier and Stefan Toepler. New York: Springer.

Glennie, Jonathan, and Andy Sumner. 2016. *Aid, Growth and Democracy*. London: Palgrave Pivot.

Glewwe, Paul, Nauman Ilias, and Michael Kremer. 2010. "Teacher Incentives." *International Encyclopedia of Education* 2: 481–488.

Goertz, Gary. 2006. *Social Science Concepts: A User's Guide*. Princeton: Princeton University Press.

Goetz, Anne Marie, and John Gaventa. 2001. "Bringing Citizen Voice and Client Focus into Service Delivery." IDS Working Paper 138, Institute of Development Studies, Brighton, UK.

Goetz, Anne Marie, and Rob Jenkins. 2001. "Hybrid Forms of Accountability: Citizen Engagement in Institutions of Public-Sector Oversight in India." *Public Management Review* 3 (3): 363–383.

Goetz, Anne Marie, and Rob Jenkins. 2005. *Reinventing Accountability: Making Democracy Work for Human Development*. Basingstoke, UK: Palgrave Macmillan.

Gomanee, Karuna, Oliver Morrissey, Paul Mosley, and Arjan Verschoor. 2005. "Aid, Government Expenditure, and Aggregate Welfare." *World Development* 33 (3): 355–370.

Gouldner, A. W. 1960. "The Norm of Reciprocity: A Preliminary Statement." *American Sociological Review* 25 (2): 161–178.

Grandvoinnet, Helene, Ghazia Aslam, and Shomikho Raha. 2015. *Opening the Black Box: The Contextual Drivers of Social Accountability*. New York: International Bank for Reconstruction and Development/World Bank.

Granovetter, Mark S. 1973. "The Strength of Weak Ties." *American Journal of Sociology* 78 (6): 1360–1380.

Graves, Casey M., Annie Haakenstad, and Joseph L. Dieleman. 2015. "Tracking Development Assistance for Health to Fragile States: 2005–2011." *Globalization and Health* 11 (1): 1–7.

Grimes, Marcia. 2013. "The Contingencies of Societal Accountability: Examining the Link Between Civil Society and Good Government." *Studies in Comparative International Development* 48 (4): 380–402.

Grootaert, Christiaan, and Thierry van Bastelaer, eds. 2002. *The Role of Social Capital in Development: An Empirical Assessment*. Cambridge, UK: Cambridge University Press.

Guillaumont, Patrick, and Rachid Laajaj. 2006. "When Instability Increases the Effectiveness of Aid Projects." Policy Research Working Papers 4034, World Bank, Washington DC.

Haines, Andy, David Sanders, Uta Lehmann, et al. 2007. "Achieving Child Survival Goals: Potential Contribution of Community Health Workers." *Lancet* 369 (9579): 2121–2131.

Han, Hahrie C. 2009. Moved to Action. Stanford: Stanford University Press.

Haq, Mahbub ul. 1995. *Reflections on Human Development*. Oxford: Oxford University Press.

Hardin, Garrett. 1968. "The Tragedy of the Commons." *Science* 162 (3859): 1243–1248.

Harris, Adam S., and Erin Hern. 2018. "Taking to the Streets: Protest as an Expression of Political Preference in Africa." *Comparative Political Studies* 52 (2): 29–31.

Heckman, James J. 1979. "Sample Selection Bias as a Specification Error." *Econometrica* 47 (1): 153–161.

Helliwell, John F., and Robert D. Putnam. 2004. "The Social Context of Well-Being." *Philosophical Transactions of the Royal Society of London. Series B: Biological Sciences* 359: 1435–1446.

Hellmeier, Sebastian, and Michael Bernhard. 2023. "Regime Transformation from Below: Mobilization for Democracy and Autocracy from 1900 to 2019." *Comparative Political Studies* 56 (12): 1858–1890.

Helmke, Gretchen, and Steven Levitsky. 2004. "Informal Institutions and Comparative Politics: A Research Agenda." *Perspectives on Politics* 2 (4): 725–740.

Hernández, Alison, Anna Karin Hurtig, Isabel Goicolea, et al. 2020. "Building Collective Power in Citizen-Led Initiatives for Health Accountability in Guatemala: The Role of Networks." *BMC Health Services Research* 20 (416): 1–14.

Hernández, Alison, Ana Lorena Ruano, Anna Karin Hurtig, Isabel Goicolea, Miguel San Sebastián, and Walter Flores. 2019. "Pathways to Accountability in Rural Guatemala: A Qualitative Comparative Analysis of Citizen-Led Initiatives for the Right to Health of Indigenous Populations." *World Development* 113: 392–401.

Hickey, Sam, and Sophie King. 2016. "Understanding Social Accountability: Politics, Power and Building New Social Contracts." *Journal of Development Studies* 52 (8): 1225–1240.

Hirschman, Albert O. 1970. *Exit, Voice, and Loyalty: Responses to Decline in Firms, Organizations, and State.* Cambridge, MA: Harvard University Press.

HNPS. 2014. "Health Nutrition and Population Statistics." National Health Account database, World Bank. https://databank.worldbank.org/source/health-nutrition -and-population-statistics.

Hoeffler, Anke, and Verity Outram. 2011. "Need, Merit, or Self-Interest—What Determines the Allocation of Aid?" *Review of Development Economics* 15 (2): 237–250.

Hoffman, Michael, and Amaney Jamal. 2014. "Religion in the Arab Spring: Between Two Competing Narratives." *Journal of Politics* 76 (3): 593–606.

Honaker, James, and Gary King. 2010. "What to Do About Missing Values in Time-Series Cross-Section Data." *American Journal of Political Science* 54 (2): 561–581.

Hooghe, Marc, and Dietlind Stolle. 2003. "Introduction: Generating Social Capital." In *Generating Social Capital: Civil Society and Institutions in Comparative Perspective*, edited by Marc Hooghe and Dietlind Stolle. New York: Palgrave Macmillan.

Howard, Marc Morjé. 2003. *The Weakness of Civil Society in Post-Communist Europe.* Cambridge, UK: Cambridge University Press.

Hsiao, Allan J., and Connor A. Emdin. 2015. "The Association Between Development Assistance for Health and Malaria, HIV and Tuberculosis Mortality: A Cross-National Analysis." *Journal of Epidemiology and Global Health* 5 (1): 41–48.

Hsiao, William C. L., and Yuanli Liu. 1996. "Economic Reform and Health: Lessons from China." *New England Journal of Medicine* 335 (6): 430–432.

Hughes, Melanie M., Pamela Paxton, Sharon Quinsaat, and Nicholas Reith. 2018. "Does the Global North Still Dominate Women's International Organizing? A Network Analysis from 1978 to 2008." *Mobilization* 23 (1): 1–21. https://doi.org/10.17813/1086 -671X-23-1-1.

Huntington, Samuel P. 1968. *Political Order in Changing Societies*. New Haven, CT: Yale University Press.

IHME. 2015. "Financing Global Health 2014: Shifts in Funding as the MDG Era Closes." Institute for Health Metrics and Evaluation, Seattle.

IHME. 2016. "Financing Global Health: Visualization Hub." Institute for Health Metrics and Evaluation, Seattle. Accessed December 4, 2016. https://vizhub.healthdata.org /fgh/.

IHME. 2017. "Development Assistance for Health Database 1990–2016." Institute for Health Metrics and Evaluation, Seattle.

Inglehart, R., C. Haerpfer, A. Moreno, et al., eds. 2014. World Values Survey: All Rounds—Country-Pooled Datafile, Dataset Version 3.0.0, JD Systems Institute and WVSA Secretariat, Madrid and Vienna. https://www.worldvaluessurvey.org /WVSDocumentationWVL.jsp.

Inglehart, Ronald F., and Christian Welzel. 2005. *Modernization, Cultural Change, and Democracy: The Human Development Sequence*. Cambridge, UK: Cambridge University Press.

Inkeles, Alex. 2000. "Measuring Social Capital and Its Consequences." *Policy Sciences* 33: 245–268.

Isaac, T. M. Thomas, and Patrick Heller. 2003. "Democracy and Development: Decentralized Planning in Kerala." In *Deepening Democracy: Institutional Innovations in Empowered Participatory Governance*, edited by Archon Fung and Erik Olin Wright. London: Verso.

ISD. 2013. "Indices of Social Development." International Institute of Social Studies, Erasmus University, Rotterdam. https://isd.iss.nl/data-access/.

Isham, Jonathan, and Satu Kähkönen. 2002. "Institutional Determinants of the Impact of Community-Based Water Services: Evidence from Sri Lanka and India." *Economic Development and Cultural Change* 50 (3): 667–691.

Isham, Jonathan, Daniel Kaufmann, and Lant Pritchett. 1997. "Civil Liberties, Democracy, and the Performance of Government Projects." *World Bank Economic Review* 11 (2): 219–242.

Isham, Jonathan, Deepa Narayan, and Lant Pritchett. 1995. "Does Participation Improve Performance? Establishing Causality with Subjective Data." *World Bank Economic Review* 9 (2): 175–200.

Ishihara, Hiroe, and Unai Pascual. 2009. "Social Capital in Community Level Environmental Governance: A Critique." *Ecological Economics* 68 (5): 1549–1562.

Jamal, Amaney A. 2009. *Barriers to Democracy: The Other Side of Social Capital in Palestine and the Arab World*. Princeton: Princeton University Press.

Jiménez-Rubio, Dolores. 2014. "Fiscal Decentralizing of Health Services." In *Decentralizing Health Services*, edited by Krishna Regmi. New York: Springer.

Joshi, Anuradha. 2013. "Do They Work? Assessing the Impact of Transparency and Accountability Initiatives in Service Delivery." *Development Policy Review* 31 (S1): 29–48.

Joshi, Anuradha. 2023. "What Makes 'Difficult' Settings Difficult? Contextual Challenges for Accountability." *Development Policy Review* 41 (S1): 1–19.

Jylhä, Marja. 2009. "What Is Self-Rated Health and Why Does It Predict Mortality? Towards a Unified Conceptual Model." *Social Science and Medicine* 69 (3): 307–316.

Kähkönen, Satu. 1999. "Does Social Capital Matter in Water and Sanitation Delivery?" Social Capital Initiative Working Paper no. 9, World Bank, Washington, DC.

Kakietek, Jakub, Tesfayi Geberselassie, Brigitte Manteuffel, et al. 2013. "It Takes a Village: Community-Based Organizations and the Availability and Utilization of HIV/AIDS-Related Services in Nigeria." *AIDS Care* 25 (Suppl. 1): S78–S87.

Kalyvitis, Sarantis, and Irene Vlachaki. 2010. "Democratic Aid and the Democratization of Recipients." *Contemporary Economic Policy* 28 (2): 188–218.

Kalyvitis, Sarantis, and Irene Vlachaki. 2012. "When Does More Aid Imply Less Democracy? An Empirical Examination." *European Journal of Political Economy* 28 (1): 132–146.

Kang, Jiyoung. 2010. "Understanding Non-Governmental Organizations in Community Development: Strengths, Limitations and Suggestions." *International Social Work* 54 (2): 223–237.

Kanyinga, Karuti. 2010. "Civil Society and Social Capital in East Africa." In *International Encyclopedia of Civil Society*, edited by Helmut Anheier and Stefan Toepler. New York: Springer.

Karatnycky, Adrian, ed. 1999. *Freedom in the World: The Annual Survey of Political Rights and Civil Liberties 1998–1999.* New York: Freedom House.

Karatnycky, Adrian, ed. 2000. *Freedom in the World: The Annual Survey of Political Rights and Civil Liberties 1999–2000.* New York: Freedom House.

Kaufmann, Daniel, Aart Kraay, and Massimo Mastruzzi. 2011. "The Worldwide Governance Indicators: Methodology and Analytical Issues." *Hague Journal on the Rule of Law* 3 (2): 220–246.

Kawachi, Ichiro, Bruce P. Kennedy, and Roberta Glass. 1999. "Social Capital and Self-Rated Health: A Contextual Analysis." *American Journal of Public Health* 89 (8): 1187–1193.

Kawachi, Ichiro, S. V. Subramanian, and Daniel Kim. 2008. *Social Capital and Health.* New York: Springer.

Keefer, Philip, and Stuti Khemani. 2016. "The Government Response to Informed Citizens: New Evidence on Media Access and the Distribution of Public Health Benefits in Africa." *World Bank Economic Review* 30 (2): 233–267.

Keohane, Robert, and Ruth Grant. 2005. "Accountability and Abuses of Power in World Politics." *American Political Science Review* 99 (1): 29–43.

Kew, Darren, and Modupe Oshikoya. 2014. "Escape from Tyranny: Civil Society and Democratic Struggle in Africa." In *The Handbook of Civil Society in Africa*, edited by Ebenezer Obadare. New York: Springer.

Khwaja, Asim Ijaz. 2004. "Is Increasing Community Participation Always a Good Thing?" *Journal of the European Economic Association* 2 (2–3): 427–436.

King, Gary, Robert Keohane, and Sidney Verba. 1995. *Designing Social Inquiry: Scientific Inference in Qualitative Research.* Princeton: Princeton University Press.

Kizhakethalackal, Elsy Thomas, Debasri Mukherjee, and Eskander Alvi. 2013. "Quantile Regression Analysis of Health-Aid and Infant Mortality: A Note." *Applied Economics Letters* 20 (13): 1197–1201.

Klesner, Joseph L. 2007. "Social Capital and Political Participation in Latin America: Evidence from Argentina, Chile, Mexico." *Latin American Research Review* 42 (2): 1–32.

Klesner, Joseph L. 2009. "Who Participates? Determinants of Political Action in Mexico." *Latin American Politics and Society* 51 (2): 59–90.

Klingemann, Hans-Dieter. 2014. "Dissatisfied Democrats: Democratic Maturation in Old and New Democracies." In *The Civic Culture Revisited: From Allegiant to Assertive Citizens*, edited by Russell Dalton and Christian Welzel. Cambridge, UK: Cambridge University Press.

Knack, Stephen. 2001. "Aid Dependence and the Quality of Governance: Cross-Country Empirical Test." *Southern Economic Journal* 68 (2): 310–329.

Knack, Stephen. 2002. "Social Capital and the Quality of Government: Evidence from the States." *American Journal of Political Science* 46 (4): 772–785.

Knack, Stephen. 2004. "Does Foreign Aid Promote Democracy?" *International Studies Quarterly* 48 (1): 251–266.

Knack, Stephen, and Philip Edward Keefer. 1997. "Does Social Capital Have an Economic Payoff? A Cross-Country Investigation." *Quarterly Journal of Economics* 112 (4): 1251–1288.

Knowles, Stephen, and P. Dorian Owen. 2010. "Which Institutions Are Good for Your Health? The Deep Determinants of Comparative Cross-Country Health Status." *Journal of Development Studies* 46 (4): 701–723.

Kosack, Stephen. 2003. "Effective Aid: How Democracy Allows Development Aid to Improve the Quality of Life." *World Development* 31 (1): 1–22.

Krasner, Stephen D., and Jeremy M. Weinstein. 2014. "Improving Governance from the Outside In." *Annual Review of Political Science* 17 (1): 123–145.

Krishna, Anirudh. 2002. *Active Social Capital*. New York: Columbia University Press.

Krug, Etienne G., Linda L. Dahlberg, James A. Mercy, Anthony B. Zwi, and Rafael Lozano. 2002. *World Report on Violence and Health*. Geneva: World Health Organization.

Kruse, Stefan. 2023. "Modernization." In *Elgar Encyclopedia of Political Sociology*, edited by Maria Grasso and Marco Guigni, 301–5. Cheltenham, UK: Edward Elgar Publishing. https://doi.org/https://doi.org/10.4337/9781803921235.00083.

La Porta, Rafael, Florencio Lopez-de-Silanes, Andrei Shleifer, and Robert W. Vishny. 1997. "Trust in Large Organizations." *American Economic Review Papers and Proceedings* 87 (2): 333–338.

Lancaster, Carol. 2006. *Foreign Aid: Diplomacy, Development, Domestic Politics*. Chicago: University of Chicago Press.

Lane, Christopher, and Amanda Glassman. 2007. "Bigger and Better? Scaling Up and Innovation in Health Aid." *Health Affairs* 26 (4): 935–948.

Larsson, Fredrik, and Marcia Grimes. 2022. "Societal Accountability and Grand Corruption: How Institutions Shape Citizens' Efforts to Shape Institutions." *Political Studies* 71 (4). https://doi.org/10.1177/00323217211067134.

Lauth, Hans-Joachim. 2015. "Formal and Informal Institutions." In *Routledge Handbook of Comparative Political Institutions*, edited by Jennifer Gandhi and Rubén Ruiz-Rufino. Abingdon, UK: Routledge.

Lee, Taeku. 2011. "The (Im)possibility of Mobilizing Public Opinion?" In *Accountability Through Public Opinion: From Inertia to Public Action*, edited by Sina Odugbemi and Taeku Lee. Washington, DC: World Bank.

Lessmann, Christian, and Gunther Markwardt. 2010. "One Size Fits All? Decentralization, Corruption, and the Monitoring of Bureaucrats." *World Development* 38 (4): 631–646.

Lessmann, Christian, and Gunther Markwardt. 2012. "Aid, Growth and Devolution." *World Development* 40 (9): 1723–1749.

Lewis, David. 1998. "Development NGOs and the Challenge of Partnership: Changing Relations Between North and South." *Social Policy & Administration* 32 (5): 501–512.

Lewis, David, and Nazneen Kanji. 2009. *Non-Governmental Organizations and Development*. Abingdon, UK: Routledge.

Lieberman, Evan S., and Daniel N. Posner. 2014. "Does Information Lead to More Active Citizenship? Evidence from an Education Intervention in Rural Kenya." *World Development* 60: 69–83.

Lin, Nan. 2008. "A Network Theory of Social Capital." In *Handbook of Social Capital*, edited by Dario Castiglione, Jan van Deth, and Guglielmo Wolleb. New York: Oxford University Press.

Linz, Juan. 1978. *The Breakdown of Democratic Regimes: Crisis, Breakdown and Reequilibrium*. Baltimore: Johns Hopkins University Press.

Linz, Juan J., and Alfred Stepan. 1996. *Problems of Democratic Transition and Consolidation*. Baltimore: Johns Hopkins University Press.

Lipset, Seymour Martin. 1959. "Some Social Requisites of Democracy: Economic Development and Political Legitimacy." *American Political Science Review* 53 (1): 69–105.

Lipset, Seymour Martin. 1960. *Political Man: The Social Bases of Politics*. New York: Doubleday & Company.

Liverani, Andrea. 2010. "Civil Society and Social Capital in North Africa." In *International Encyclopedia of Civil Society*, edited by Helmut Anheier and Stefan Toepler. New York: Springer.

Lodenstein, Elsbet, Marjolein Dieleman, Barend Gerretsen, and Jacqueline E. W. Broerse. 2017. "Health Provider Responsiveness to Social Accountability Initiatives in Low- and Middle-Income Countries: A Realist Review." *Health Policy and Planning* 32 (1): 125–140.

Loewenson, Rene. 1998. "Public Participation in Health: Making People Matter." Working Paper 84, Institute of Development Studies, Brighton, UK.

Lu, Chunling, Matthew T. Schneider, Paul Gubbins, Katherine Leach-Kemon, Dean Jamison, and Christopher J. L. Murray. 2010. "Public Financing of Health in Developing Countries: A Cross-National Systematic Analysis." *Lancet* 375 (9723): 1375–1387.

Macedo, Stephen, Yvette Alex-Assensoh Fung, Jeffrey M. Berry, et al. 2005. *Democracy at Risk: How Political Choices Undermine Citizen Participation and What We Can Do About It*. Washington, DC: Brookings Institution Press.

Macinko, James, Maria de Fátima Marinho de Souza, Frederico C. Guanais, and Celso Cardoso da Silva Simões. 2007. "Going to Scale with Community-Based Primary Care: An Analysis of the Family Health Program and Infant Mortality in Brazil, 1999–2004." *Social Science and Medicine* 65 (10): 2070–2080.

Mafuta, Eric M., Marjolein A. Dieleman, Lisanne M. Hogema, et al. 2015. "Social Accountability for Maternal Health Services in Muanda and Bolenge Health

Zones, Democratic Republic of Congo: A Situation Analysis." *BMC Health Services Research* 15 (1): 1–17.

Mafuta, Eric M., Lisanne Hogema, Thérèse N. M. Mambu, et al. 2016. "Understanding the Local Context and Its Possible Influences on Shaping, Implementing and Running Social Accountability Initiatives for Maternal Health Services in Rural Democratic Republic of the Congo: A Contextual Factor Analysis." *BMC Health Services Research* 16 (640): 1–13.

Malena, Carmen, and Mary McNeil. 2010. "Social Accountability in Africa: An Introduction." In *Demanding Good Governance*, edited by Mary McNeil and Carmen Malena. Washington, DC: World Bank.

Mansuri, Ghazala. 2012. "Bottom Up or Top Down: Participation and the Provision of Local Public Goods." Brief 6. Washington, DC: World Bank–Pakistan Poverty Alleviation Fund.

Mansuri, Ghazala, and Vijayendra Rao. 2013. *Localizing Development: Does Participation Work?* Washington, DC: World Bank.

Markowski, Radoslaw. 2011. "Responsiveness." In *International Encyclopedia of Political Science*, edited by Bertrand Badie, Dirk Berg-Schlosser, and Leonardo Morlino. London: SAGE Publications.

Markus, Hazel Rose. 2016. "What Moves People to Action? Culture and Motivation." *Current Opinion in Psychology* 8: 161–166.

Markus, Hazel Rose, and Shinobu Kitayama. 1991. "Culture and the Self: Implications for Cognition, Emotion, and Motivation." *Psychological Review* 98 (2): 224–253.

Marshall, Monty G., and Gabrielle C. Elzinga-Marshall. 2017. *Global Report 2017: Conflict, Governance, and State Fragility*. USA: Center for Systemic Peace.

Marshall, Monty G., Ted Robert Gurr, and Keith Jaggers. 2014. *Polity IV Project, Political Regime Characteristics and Transitions, 1800–2014, Data*. USA: Center for Systemic Peace.

Martens, Bertin. 2002. "Evaluation." In *The Institutional Economics of Foreign Aid*, edited by Bertin Martens, Uwe Mummert, Peter Murrell, and Paul Seabright. Cambridge, UK: Cambridge University Press.

Martin, Gayle, and Obert Pimhidzai. 2013. *Service Delivery Indicators: Kenya*. Washington, DC: World Bank.

Masud, Nadia, and Boriana Yontcheva. 2005. "Does Foreign Aid Reduce Poverty? Empirical Evidence from Nongovernmental and Bilateral Aid." IMF Working Paper WP/05/100, International Monetary Fund.

McGuire, James W. 2010. *Wealth, Health, and Democracy in East Asia and Latin America*. Cambridge, UK: Cambridge University Press.

McGuire, James W. 2020. *Democracy and Population Health*. Cambridge, UK: Cambridge University Press.

Mejia, Steven Andrew. 2022. "Democracy and Health in Developing Countries: New Cross-National Evidence, 1990–2016." *Sociological Perspectives* 65 (5): 981–1000.

Michener, Jamila. 2018. *Fragmented Democracy*. Cambridge, UK: Cambridge University Press.

Miller, Nathan P., Agbessi Amouzou, Elizabeth Hazel, et al. 2016. "Assessment of the Impact of Quality Improvement Interventions on the Quality of Sick Child Care

Provided by Health Extension Workers in Ethiopia." *Journal of Global Health* 6 (2): 1–9.

Mishra, Prachi, and David Newhouse. 2009. "Does Health Aid Matter?" *Journal of Health Economics* 28 (4): 855–872.

Mogedal, Sigrun, Sissel Hodne Steen, and George Mpelumbe. 1995. "Health Sector Reform and Organization Issues at the Local Level: Lessons from Selected African Countries." *Journal of International Development* 7 (3): 349–367.

Molenaers, Nadia. 2005. "Tracing the Contradictions: Associational Life Versus Informal Networks in a Third World Context." In *Democracy and the Role of Associations*, edited by Sigrid Roßteutscher. London: Routledge.

Molenaers, Nadia, Sebastian Dellepiane, and Jörg Faust. 2015. "Political Conditionality and Foreign Aid." *World Development* 75: 2–12. https://doi.org/10.1016/j.worlddev.2015.04.001.

Molina, Ezequiel, and Gayle Martin. 2016. *Health Service Delivery in Mozambique*. Washington, DC: World Bank.

Morrissey, Oliver. 2015. "Aid and Government Fiscal Behavior: Assessing Recent Evidence." *World Development* 69: 98–105.

Mosley, Paul, and Marion J. Eeckhout. 2000. "From Project Aid to Programme Assistance." In *Foreign Aid and Development: Lessons Learnt and Directions for the Future*, edited by Finn Tarp and Peter Hjertholm. London: Routledge.

Mularidharan, Karthik, and Venkatesh Sundararaman. 2011. "Teacher Performance Pay: Experimental Evidence from India." *Journal of Political Economy* 119 (1): 39–77.

Munck, Gerardo L., and Jay Verkuilen. 2002. "Evaluating Alternative Indices." *Comparative Political Studies* 35 (1): 5–34.

Murtazashvili, Jennifer Brick. 2016. *Informal Order and the State in Afghanistan*. Cambridge, UK: Cambridge University Press.

Murtin, Fabrice. 2013. "Long-Term Determinants of the Demographic Transition, 1870–2000." *Review of Economics and Statistics* 95 (2): 617–631.

Nair, Nirmala, Prasanta Tripathy, Audrey Prost, Anthony Costello, and David Osrin. 2010. "Improving Newborn Survival in Low-Income Countries: Community-Based Approaches and Lessons from South Asia." *PLoS Medicine* 7 (4): 1–9.

Najam, Adil. 1996. "NGO Accountability: A Conceptual Framework." *Development Policy Review* 14 (4): 339–353.

Narayan, Deepa. 1995. *The Contribution of People's Participation: Evidence from 121 Rural Water Supply Projects*. Washington, DC: World Bank.

Natal, Alejandro, Jorge Cadena-Roa, and Sara Gordon Rappoport. 2010. "Civil Society and Social Capital in Mexico and Central America." In *International Encyclopedia of Civil Society*, edited by Helmut Anheier and Stefan Toepler. New York: Springer.

Newton, Kenneth. 2001. "Trust, Social Capital, Civil Society, and Democracy." *International Political Science Review* 22 (2): 201–214.

Nolan, Terry, Patria Angos, Antonia J. L. Cunha, et al. 2001. "Quality of Hospital Care for Seriously Ill Children in Less-Developed Countries." *Lancet* 357 (9250): 106–110.

Norris, Pippa. 2002. *Democratic Phoenix: Reinventing Political Activism*. Cambridge, UK: Cambridge University Press.

Norris, Pippa. 2012. *Making Democratic Governance Work: How Regimes Shape Prosperity, Welfare, and Peace.* New York: Cambridge University Press.

North, Douglass C. 1990. *Institutions, Institutional Change, and Economic Performance.* Cambridge, UK: Cambridge University Press.

O'Donnell, Guillermo. 1998. "Horizontal Accountability in New Democracies." *Journal of Democracy* 9 (3): 112–126.

O'Neil, Tammie, Marta Foresti, and Alan Hudson. 2007. *Evaluation of Citizens' Voice and Accountability: Review of the Literature and Donor Approaches Report.* London: Department for International Development (DFID).

Oakley, Peter. 1991. *Projects with People: The Practice of Participation in Rural Development.* Geneva: International Labour Organization.

Oberndörfer, Dieter, Theodor Hanf, and Heribert Weiland. 2010. *Verfahren der Wirkungsanalyse: Ein Handbuch für die Entwicklungspolitische Praxis.* Freiburg im Breisgau: Arbeitskreis "Evaluation von Entwicklungspolitik" DeGEval—Deutsche Gesellschaft für Evaluation, Arnold-Bergstraesser-Institut.

Odugbemi, Sina, and Taeku Lee, eds. 2011a. *Accountability Through Public Opinion: From Inertia to Public Action.* Washington, DC: World Bank.

Odugbemi, Sina, and Taeku Lee. 2011b. "Appendix A." In *Accountability Through Public Opinion: From Inertia to Public Action*, edited by Sina Odugbemi and Taeku Lee. Washington, DC: World Bank.

Odugbemi, Sina, and Taeku Lee. 2011c. "Taking Direct Accountability Seriously." In *Accountability Through Public Opinion: From Inertia to Public Action*, edited by Sina Odugbemi and Taeku Lee. Washington, DC: World Bank.

Olken, Benjamin A. 2007. "Monitoring Corruption: Evidence from a Field Experiment in Indonesia." *Journal of Political Economy* 115 (2): 200–249.

Olson, Mancur. 1965. *The Logic of Collective Action: Public Goods and the Theory of Groups.* Cambridge, MA: Harvard University Press.

Olson, Mancur. 1971. *The Logic of Collective Action: Public Goods and the Theory of Groups.* 2nd printing with a new preface and appendix. Cambridge, MA: Harvard University Press.

Östlin, Piroska, Asha George, and Gita Sen. 2001. "Gender, Health, and Equity: The Intersections." In *Challenging Inequities in Health: From Ethics to Action*, edited by Timothy Evans, Margaret Whitehead, Finn Diderichsen, Abbas Bhuiya, and Meg Wirth. New York: Oxford University Press.

Ostrom, Elinor. 1990. *Governing the Commons: The Evolution of Institutions for Collective Action.* Cambridge, UK: Cambridge University Press.

Ostrom, Elinor. 1996. "Crossing the Great Divide: Coproduction, Synergy, and Development." *World Development* 24 (6): 1073–1087.

Ostrom, Elinor. 1999. "Coping with Tragedies of the Commons." *Annual Review of Political Science* 2 (1): 493–535.

Ostrom, Elinor, and T. K. Ahn. 2008. "Social Capital and Collective Action." In *The Handbook of Social Capital*, edited by Dario Castiglione, Jan van Deth, and Guglielmo Wolleb. New York: Oxford University Press.

Paul, Samuel. 1992. "Accountability in Public Services: Exit, Voice and Control." *World Development* 20 (7): 1047–1060.

Paxton, Pamela. 2002. "Social Capital and Democracy: An Interdependent Relationship." *American Sociological Review* 67 (2): 254–277.

Paxton, Pamela. 2007. "Association Memberships and Generalized Trust: A Multilevel Model Across 31 Countries." *Social Forces* 86 (1): 47–76.

Paxton, Pamela, Melanie M. Hughes, and Jennifer L. Green. 2006. "The International Women's Movement and Women's Political Representation, 1893–2003." *American Sociological Review* 71 (6): 898–920.

Paxton, Pamela, Melanie M. Hughes, and Nicholas E. Reith. 2015. "Extending the INGO Network Country Score, 1950–2008." *Sociological Science* 2: 287–307. https://doi.org/10.15195/v2.a14.

Paxton, Pamela, and Robert W. Ressler. 2017. "Trust and Participation in Associations." In *The Oxford Handbook of Social and Political Trust*, edited by Eric M. Uslaner. Oxford: Oxford University Press.

Pemstein, Daniel, Kyle L. Marquardt, Eitan Tzelgov, Yi-ting Wang, and Farhad Miri. 2015. "The Varieties of Democracy Measurement Model: Latent Variable Analysis for Cross-National and Cross-Temporal Expert-Coded Data." V-Dem Working Paper Series 2015:21, Varieties of Democracy Institute, Gothenburg, Sweden.

Persson, Anna, Bo Rothstein, and Jan Teorell. 2013. "Why Anticorruption Reforms Fail—Systemic Corruption as a Collective Action Problem." *Governance* 26 (3): 449–471.

Peruzzotti, Enrique. 2011. "The Workings of Accountability: Contexts and Conditions." In *Accountability Through Public Opinion: From Inertia to Public Action*, edited by Sina Odugbemi and Taeku Lee. Washington, DC: World Bank.

Platteau, Jean Philippe. 2004. "Monitoring Elite Capture in Community-Driven Development." *Development and Change* 35 (2): 223–246.

Portes, Alejandro. 2000. "The Two Meanings of Social Capital." *Sociological Forum* 15 (1): 1–12.

Poullier, Jean Pierre, Patricia Hernandez, and Kei Kawabata. 2002. "National Health Accounts: Concepts, Data Sources and Methodology." Evidence and Information for Policy Cluster (EIP) Discussion Paper Series: WHO/EIP/02.47, World Health Organization, Geneva.

Pretty, Jules N. 1995. "Participatory Learning for Sustainable Agriculture." *World Development* 23 (8): 1247–1263.

Pritchett, Lant, Michael Woolcock, and Matt Andrews. 2013. "Looking like a State: Techniques of Persistent Failure in State Capability for Implementation." *Journal of Development Studies* 49 (1): 1–18.

Prud'homme, Rémy. 1995. "The Dangers of Decentralization." *World Bank Research Observer* 10 (2): 201–220.

Putnam, Robert D. 1993. *Making Democracy Work: Civic Traditions in Modern Italy*. New Jersey: Princeton University Press.

Putnam, Robert D. 1995. "Tuning In, Tuning Out: The Strange Disappearance of Social Capital in America." *Political Science & Politics* 28: 664–683.

Putnam, Robert D. 2000. *Bowling Alone: The Collapse and Revival of American Community*. New York: Simon & Schuster.

Rajan, Raghuram G., and Arvind Subramanian. 2007. "Does Aid Affect Governance?" *American Economic Review* 97 (2): 322–327.

Rajan, Raghuram G., and Arvind Subramanian. 2008. "Aid and Growth: What Does the Cross-Country Evidence Really Show?" *Review of Economics and Statistics* 90 (4): 643–665.

Rao, Vijayendra, and Ana María Ibáñez. 2005. "The Social Impact of Social Funds in Jamaica: A 'Participatory Econometric' Analysis of Targeting, Collective Action, and Participation in Community-Driven Development." *Journal of Development Studies* 41 (5): 788–838.

Rauch, James E., and Peter B. Evans. 2000. "Bureaucratic Structure and Bureaucratic Performance in Less Developed Countries." *Journal of Public Economics* 75 (1): 49–71.

Riddell, Roger C. 2013. "Assessing the Overall Impact of Civil Society on Development at the Country Level: An Exploratory Approach." *Development Policy Review* 31 (4): 371–396.

Riehman, Kara S., Jakub Kakietek, Brigitte A. Manteuffel, et al. 2013. "Evaluating the Effects of Community-Based Organization Engagement on HIV and AIDS-Related Risk Behavior in Kenya." *AIDS Care* 25 (Suppl. 1): 67–77.

Riker, W. H. 1964. *Federalism: Origin, Operation, Significance.* Boston: Little Brown.

Risse, Thomas, Tanja A. Börzel, and Anke Draude, eds. 2018. *The Oxford Handbook of Governance and Limited Statehood.* Oxford: Oxford University Press.

Rocha Menocal, Alina, and Bhavna Sharma. 2008. *Joint Evaluation of Citizens' Voice and Accountability: Synthesis Report.* London: Department for International Development (DFID).

Rockmore, Christophe. 2016. *Health Service Delivery in Togo.* Washington, DC: World Bank.

Roitter, Mario. 2010. "Civil Society and Social Capital in South America." In *International Encyclopedia of Civil Society*, edited by Helmut Anheier and Stefan Toepler. New York: Springer.

Roller, Edeltraud. 2005. *The Performance of Democracies: Political Institutions and Public Policy.* Oxford: Oxford University Press.

Roodman, David. 2008. "Through the Looking-Glass, and What OLS Found There: On Growth, Foreign Aid, and Reverse Causality." Center for Global Development Working Paper no. 137, Center for Global Development, Washington, DC.

Roodman, David. 2009. "How to Do xtabond2: An Introduction to Difference and System GMM in Stata." *Stata Journal* 9 (1): 86–136.

Roodman, David. 2014. "The Impact of Life-Saving Interventions on Fertility." David Roodman (website). http://davidroodman.com/blog/2014/04/16/the-mortality-fertility-link/.

Roßteutscher, Sigrid. 2010. "Social Capital Worldwide: Potential for Democratization or Stabilizer of Authoritarian Rule?" *American Behavioral Scientist* 53 (5): 737–757.

Rothstein, Bo, and Rasmus Broms. 2012. "Social Capital." In *Routledge Handbook of Democratization*, edited by Jeffrey Haynes. Abingdon, UK: Routledge.

Rothstein, Bo, and Dietlind Stolle. 2008. "The State and Social Capital: An Institutional Theory of Generalized Trust." *Comparative Politics* 40 (4): 441–459.

Rothstein, Bo, and Jan Teorell. 2008. "What Is Quality of Government? A Theory of Impartial Government Institutions." *Governance* 21 (2): 165–190.

Rothstein, Bo, and Jan Teorell. 2012. "Defining and Measuring Quality of Government." In *Good Government: The Relevance of Political Science*, edited by Sören Holmberg and Bo Rothstein. Cheltenham, UK: Edward Elgar Publishing.

Saber, Alaa. 2010. "Civil Society and Social Capital in the Middle East." In *International Encyclopedia of Civil Society*, edited by Helmut Anheier and Stefan Toepler. New York: Springer.

Salehyan, Idean, Cullen S. Hendrix, Jesse Hamner, et al. 2012. "Social Conflict in Africa: A New Database." *International Interactions* 38 (4): 503–511.

Schaaf, Marta, Shruti Chhabra, Walter Flores, Francesa Feruglio, Jashodhara Dasgupta, and Ana Lorena Ruano. 2018. "Does Information and Communication Technology Add Value to Citizen-Led Accountability Initiatives in Health? Experiences from India and Guatemala." *Health and Human Rights* 20 (2): 169–184.

Schäferhoff, Marco. 2014. "External Actors and the Provision of Public Health Services in Somalia." *Governance* 27 (4): 675–695.

Schedler, Andreas, Larry Diamond, and Marc F. Plattner, eds. 1999. *The Self-Restraining State: Power and Accountability in New Democracies*. London: Boulder.

Schulz, Jonathan F., Duman Bahrami-Rad, Jonathan P. Beauchamp, and Joseph Henrich. 2019. "The Church, Intensive Kinship, and Global Psychological Variation." *Science* 366 (707): 1–12.

Segall, Malcolm. 2003. "District Health Systems in a Neoliberal World: A Review of Key Policy Areas." *International Journal of Health Planning and Management* 18: 5–26.

Seligson, Mitchell A. 1980. "Trust Efficacy and Modes of Political Participation: A Study of Costa Rican Peasants." *British Journal of Political Science* 10 (1): 75–98.

Sen, Amartyá. 1999. *Development as Freedom*. New York: Alfred Knopf.

Sheikh, Kabir, Michael Kent Ranson, and Lucy Gilson. 2014. "Explorations on People Centredness in Health Systems." *Health Policy and Planning* 29: II1–5.

Skocpol, Theda, Marshall Ganz, and Ziad Munson. 2000. "A Nation of Organizers: The Institutional Origins of Civic Voluntarism in the United States." *American Political Science Review* 94 (3): 527–546.

Speer, Johanna. 2012. "Participatory Governance Reform: A Good Strategy for Increasing Government Responsiveness and Improving Public Services?" *World Development* 40 (12): 2379–2398.

Starfield, Barbara, Leiyu Shi, and James Macinko. 2005. "Contribution of Primary Care to Health Systems and Health." *Milbank Quarterly* 83 (3): 457–502.

Stokes, Susan C. 2013. "Political Clientelism." In *The Oxford Handbook of Comparative Politics*, edited by Robert E. Goodin. Oxford: Oxford University Press.

Stolle, Dietlind. 2002. "Trusting Strangers—The Concept of Generalized Trust in Perspective." *Österreichische Zeitschrift für Politikwissenschaft* 31 (4): 397–412.

Stolle, Dietlind, and Marc Morjé Howard. 2008. "Civic Engagement and Civic Attitudes in Cross-National Perspective: Introduction to the Symposium." *Political Studies* 56 (1): 1–11.

Stuckler, David, Martin McKee, and Sanjay Basu. 2013. "Six Concerns About the Data in Aid Debates: Applying an Epidemiological Perspective to the Analysis of Aid Effectiveness in Health and Development." *Health Policy and Planning* 28 (8): 871–883.

Svensson, Jakob. 1999. "Aid, Growth and Democracy." *Economics & Politics* 11 (3): 275–297.

Tadros, Mariz. 2020. *Eleven Recommendations for Working on Empowerment and Accountability in Fragile, Conflict or Violence-Affected Settings*. Brighton, UK: Institute of Development Studies.

Talhelm, Thomas, X. Zhang, S. Oishi, et al. 2014. "Large-Scale Psychological Differences Within China Explained by Rice Versus Wheat Agriculture." *Science* 344 (May): 603–608.

Tanzi, Vito. 1996. "Fiscal Federalism and Decentralization: A Review of Some Efficiency and Macroeconomic Aspects." In *Annual World Bank Conference on Development Economics 1995*, edited by Michael Bruno and Boris Pleskovic. Washington, DC: World Bank.

Tarrow, Sidney. 1996. "Making Social Science Work Across Space and Time: A Critical Reflection on Robert Putnam's Making Democracy Work." *American Political Science Review* 90 (2): 389–397.

Tavares, José. 2003. "Does Foreign Aid Corrupt?" *Economics Letters* 79: 99–106.

Tavits, M. 2006. "Making Democracy Work More? Exploring the Linkage Between Social Capital and Government Performance." *Political Research Quarterly* 59 (2): 211–225.

Tendler, Judith. 1995. *Social Capital and the Public Sector: The Blurred Boundaries Between Private and Public*. Cambridge, MA: Massachusetts Institute of Technology.

Teorell, Jan, Nicholas Charron, Stefan Dahlberg, et al. 2013. *The Quality of Government Dataset, Version 15May13*. Gothenburg, Sweden: Quality of Government Institute. https://www.qogdata.pol.gu.se/dataarchive/codebook_standard_15may13.pdf.

Teorell, Jan, Stefan Dahlberg, Sören Holmberg, Bo Rothstein, Natalia Alvarado Pachon, and Richard Svensson. 2018. *The QOG Standard Dataset 2018, Codebook*. Gothenburg, Sweden: Quality of Government Institute.

Thirlwall, Anthony Philip. 1989. *Growth and Development: With Special Reference to Developing Economies*. 4th ed. Basingstoke, UK: Macmillan Education.

Thomas, Catherine Cole, and Hazel Rose Markus. 2023. "Enculturating the Science of International Development: Beyond the WEIRD Independent Paradigm." *Journal of Cross-Cultural Psychology* 54 (2): 195–214.

Thomson, Robert, Masaki Yuki, Thomas Talhelm, et al. 2018. "Relational Mobility Predicts Social Behaviors in 39 Countries and Is Tied to Historical Farming and Threat." *Proceedings of the National Academy of Sciences of the United States of America* 115 (29): 7521–7526.

Tierney, Michael J., Daniel L. Nielson, Darren G. Hawkins, et al. 2011. "More Dollars than Sense: Refining Our Knowledge of Development Finance Using AidData." *World Development* 39 (11): 1891–1906.

Tilly, Charles. 2006. *Regimes and Repertoires*. Chicago: University of Chicago Press.

Tilly, Charles, and Sidney Tarrow. 2015. *Contentious Politics*. Oxford: Oxford University Press.

Tulchinsky, Theodore H., and Elena A. Varavikova. 2009. *The New Public Health*. 3rd ed. San Diego: Elsevier Academic Press.

Turner, Erin L., Katie R. Nielsen, Shelina M. Jamal, Amelie von Saint André-von Arnim, and Ndidiamaka L. Musa. 2016. "A Review of Pediatric Critical Care in Resource-Limited Settings: A Look at Past, Present, and Future Directions." *Frontiers in Pediatrics* 4 (5): 1–15.

Tusalem, Rollin F. 2007. "A Boon or a Bane? The Role of Civil Society in Third- and Fourth-Wave Democracies." *International Political Science Review* 28 (3): 361–386.

Uchimura, Hiroko, and Johannes P. Jütting. 2009. "Fiscal Decentralization, Chinese Style: Good for Health Outcomes?" *World Development* 37 (12): 1926–1934.

UNDP. 1993. *Human Development Report 1993*. Oxford: Oxford University Press.

UNDP. 1997. *Decentralized Governance Programme: Strengthening Capacity for People-Centred Development*. Management Development and Governance Division. New York: United Nations Development Programme.

Uphoff, Norman. 1992. *Possibilities for Participatory Development and Post-Newtonian Social Science*. Ithaca, NY: Cornell University Press.

Van de Sijpe, Nicolas. 2012. "Is Foreign Aid Fungible? Evidence from the Education and Health Sectors." *World Bank Economic Review* 27 (2): 1–37.

Van de Sijpe, Nicolas. 2013. "The Fungibility of Health Aid Reconsidered." *Journal of Development Studies* 49 (12): 1746–1754.

Van Deth, Jan. 2016. "What Is Political Participation?" In *Oxford Research Encyclopedia of Politics*, edited by William R. Thompson. Oxford: Oxford University Press.

Van Rooy, Alison, ed. 2013. *Civil Society and the Aid Industry*. Routledge.

Varraich, Aiysha. 2014. "Corruption: An Umbrella Concept." QOG Working Papers Series 2014:04, Quality of Government Institute, Gothenburg, Sweden.

Verba, Sidney, and Norman H. Nie. 1972. *Participation in America: Political Democracy and Social Equality*. New York: Harper and Row.

Verba, Sidney, Norman H. Nie, and Jae-on Kim. 1971. *The Modes of Democratic Participation: A Cross-National Comparison*. Beverly Hills: SAGE Publications.

Verba, Sidney, Kay Lehman Schlozman, and Henry E. Brady. 1995. *Voice and Equality: Civic Volunteerism in American Politics*. Cambridge, MA: Harvard University Press.

Verba, Sidney, Kay Lehman Schlozman, Henry E. Brady, and Norman H. Nie. 1993. "Citizen Activity: Who Participates? What Do They Say?" *American Political Science Review* 87 (2): 303–318.

Walsh, Julia A., and Kenneth S. Warren. 1979. "Selective Primary Health Care: An Interim Strategy for Disease Control in Developing Countries." *New England Journal of Medicine* 301 (18): 967–974.

Walzer, Michael. 1998. "The Idea of Civil Society: A Path to Social Reconstruction." In *Community Works: The Revival of Civil Society in America*, edited by E. J. Dionne. Washington, DC: Brookings Institution Press.

Wane, Waly, and Gayle Martin. 2016. *Health Service Delivery in Uganda*. Washington, DC: World Bank.

Warren, Mark E. 2008. "The Nature and Logic of Bad Social Capital." In *The Handbook of Social Capital*, edited by Dario Castiglione, Jan van Deth, and Guglielmo Wolleb. New York: Oxford University Press.

Weber, Max. 1947. *The Theory of Social and Economic Organization*. Edited by A. M. Henderson and Talcott Parsons. New York: The Free Press.

Weber, Max. 1978. *Economy and Society*. Edited by Guenther Roth and Claus Wittich. Berkeley: University of California Press.

Weiss, Meredith. 2010. "Civil Society and Social Capital in Southeast Asia." In *International Encyclopedia of Civil Society*, edited by Helmut Anheier and Stefan Toepler. New York: Springer.

Welzel, Christian. 2013. *Freedom Rising: Human Empowerment and the Quest for Emancipation*. New York: Cambridge University Press.

Welzel, Christian. 2014. "Evolution, Empowerment, and Emancipation: How Societies Climb the Freedom Ladder." *World Development* 64 (December): 33–51.

Welzel, Christian, and Amy C. Alexander. 2017. "The Myth of Deconsolidation: Rising Liberalism and the Populist Reaction." *Journal of Democracy*. "Online Exchange on 'Democratic Deconsolidation.'" https://www.journalofdemocracy.org/online-exchange-democratic-deconsolidation/.

Welzel, Christian, and Franziska Deutsch. 2012. "Emancipative Values and Nonviolent Protest: The Importance of 'Ecological' Effects." *British Journal of Political Science* 42 (2): 465–479.

Welzel, Christian, Ronald F. Inglehart, and Franziska Deutsch. 2005. "Social Capital, Voluntary Associations and Collective Action: Which Aspects of Social Capital Have the Greatest Civic Payoff?" *Journal of Civil Society* 1 (2): 121–146.

Welzel, Christian, Ronald F. Inglehart, and Hans-Dieter Klingemann. 2003. "The Theory of Human Development: A Cross-Cultural Analysis." *European Journal of Political Research* 42: 341–379.

Welzel, Christian, Ronald F. Inglehart, and Stefan Kruse. 2017. "Pitfalls in the Study of Democratization: Testing the Emancipatory Theory of Democracy." *British Journal of Political Science* 47 (2): 463–472.

Welzel, Christian, Stefan Kruse, Steven Brieger, and Lennart Brunkert. 2025. *The COOL WATER Effect: Geo-Climatic Sources of Western Exceptionalism*. London and New York: Palgrave-MacMillan.

Wetterberg, Anna, Derick W. Brinkerhoff, and Jana C. Hertz, eds. 2016. *Governance and Service Delivery: Practical Applications of Social Accountability Across Sectors*. Durham, NC: RTI Press.

Whitaker, Gordon P. 1980. "Coproduction: Citizen Participation in Service Delivery." *Public Administration Review* 40 (3): 240–246.

WHO. 1978. Declaration of Alma-Ata, International Conference on Primary Health Care, Alma-Ata, USSR.

WHO. 2000. *The World Health Report 2000—Health Systems: Improving Performance*. Geneva: World Health Organization (WHO).

WHO. 2003. *Adherence to Long-Term Therapies: Evidence for Action*. Geneva: World Health Organization (WHO).

WHO. 2014. *World Health Statistics 2014*. Geneva: World Health Organization (WHO).

Williamson, Claudia R. 2008. "Foreign Aid and Human Development: The Impact of Foreign Aid to the Health Sector." *Southern Economic Journal* 75 (1): 188–207.

Wilson, Sven E. 2011. "Chasing Success: Health Sector Aid and Mortality." *World Development* 39 (11): 2032–2043.

Winters, Matthew. 2010. "Accountability, Participation and Foreign Aid Effectiveness." *International Studies Review* 12 (2): 218–243.

Winters, Matthew, and Gina Martinez. 2015. "The Role of Governance in Determining Foreign Aid Flow Composition." *World Development* 66: 516–531.

Woolcock, Michael. 1998. "Social Capital and Economic Development: Toward a Theoretical Synthesis and Policy Framework." *Theory and Society* 27: 151–208.

Woolcock, Michael. 2010. "The Rise and Routinization of Social Capital, 1988–2008." *Annual Review of Political Science* 13 (1): 469–487.

Woolcock, Michael. 2011. "Civil Society and Social Capital." In *Oxford Handbook of Civil Society*, edited by Michael Edwards. Oxford: Oxford University Press.

Woolcock, Michael, and Deepa Narayan. 2000. "Social Capital: Implications for Development Theory, Research, and Policy." *World Bank Research Observer* 15 (2): 225–249.

Wooldridge, Jeffrey M. 2013. *Introductory Econometrics: A Modern Approach*. 5th ed. Mason: South-Western Cengage Learning.

World Bank. 1994. *The World Bank and Participation*. Washington, DC: World Bank Operations Policy Department.

World Bank. 1998. "The Initiative on Defining, Monitoring and Measuring Social Capital: Overview and Program Description." Social Capital Initiative Working Paper 1, World Bank, Washington, DC.

World Bank. 1999. *Entering the 21st Century: World Development Report 1999/2000*. Washington, DC: Oxford University Press.

World Bank. 2000. "Mainstreaming Participation in Development." OED Working Paper Series No. 10, World Bank, Washington, DC.

World Bank. 2003. *Making Services Work for Poor People: World Development Report 2004*. Washington, DC: Oxford University Press.

World Bank. 2012. "Service Delivery Indicators in Tanzania." Service Delivery Indicators Initiative, Washington, DC.

World Bank. 2014. *Strategic Framework for Mainstreaming Citizen Engagement in World Bank Group Operations*. Washington, DC: World Bank.

World Bank. 2015. "Migration and Remittances: Recent Developments and Outlook." Migration and Development Brief 24, World Bank Development Prospects Group, Washington, DC.

World Bank. 2017. "Service Delivery Indicators (SDI) Project." Service Delivery Indicators Initiative, Washington, D.C. https://datacatalog.worldbank.org/search/dataset/0042030.

World Bank. 2018. *Poverty and Shared Prosperity 2018: Piecing Together the Poverty Puzzle*. Washington, DC: World Bank.

Wright, Joseph. 2009. "How Foreign Aid Can Foster Democratization in Authoritarian Regimes." *American Journal of Political Science* 53 (3): 552–571.

Wright, Joseph. 2010. "Aid Effectiveness and the Politics of Personalism." *Comparative Political Studies* 43 (6): 735–762.

Wright, Joseph, and Matthew Winters. 2010. "The Politics of Effective Foreign Aid." *Annual Review of Political Science* 13 (1): 61–80.

Wu, Shunquan, Rui Wang, Yanfang Zhao, et al. 2013. "The Relationship Between Self-Rated Health and Objective Health Status: A Population-Based Study." *BMC Public Health* 13 (1).

Yachkaschi, Schirin. 2010. "Civil Society and Social Capital in Central and Southern Africa." In *International Encyclopedia of Civil Society*, edited by Helmut Anheier and Stefan Toepler. New York: Springer.

Index

Online Supplement

How Ordinary People Make Aid Work is supported by an online supplement that provides figures and tables referenced in the Appendix, as well as color versions of the images in the book. The additional materials for this book can be found by visiting the specific book page on press.jhu.edu.

Appendix
Three figures and thirty tables comprise the appendix.
Appendix figure and table lists are provided on pages xiii-xvi.

Color Figures
The full collection of interior figures as generated by the author is available in color. Figure list is provided on page ix.

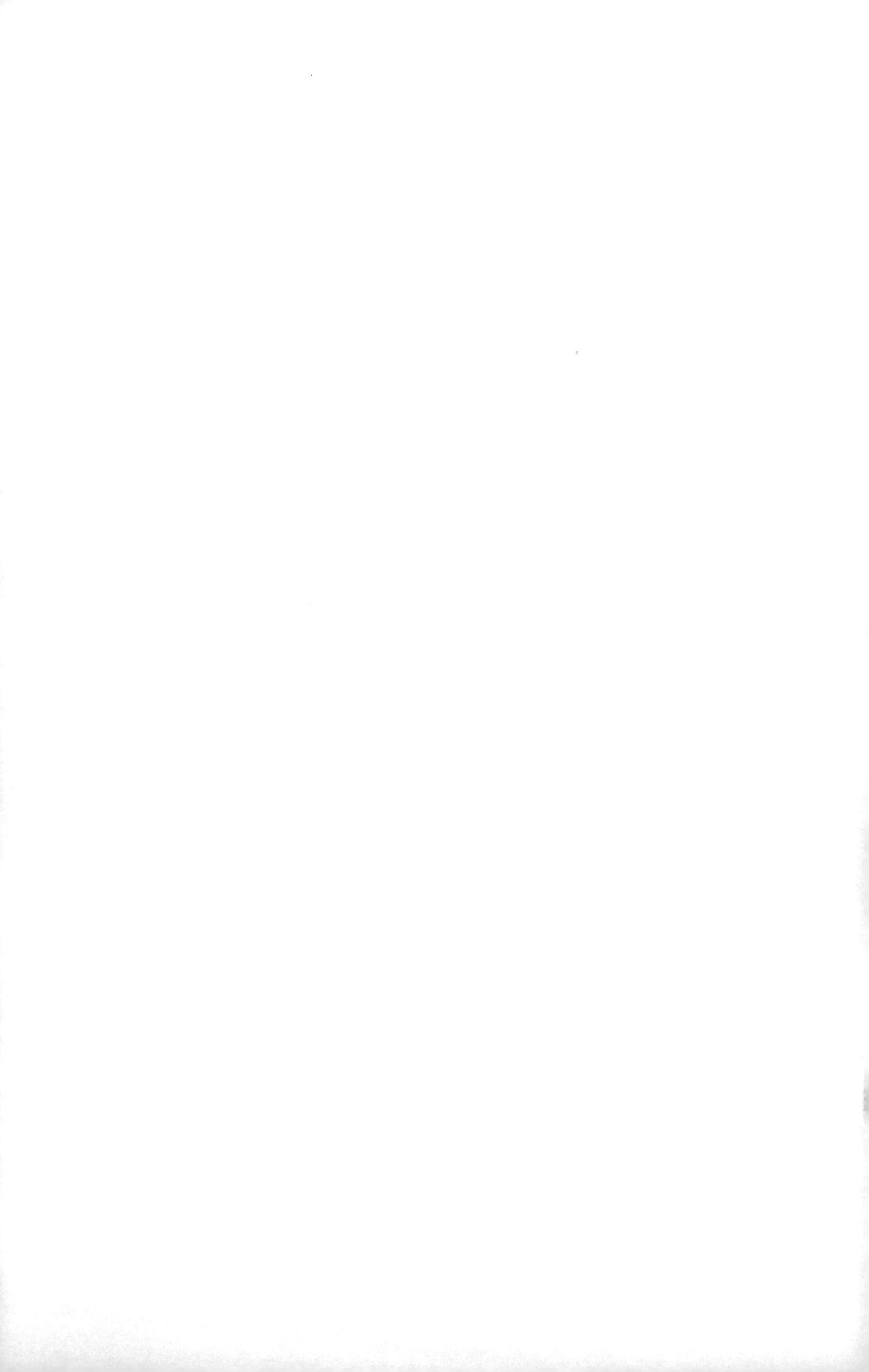